The Physiological Effects of Ageing

Implications for Nursing Practice

For Teresa, David and Shona

The Physiological Effects of Ageing

Implications for Nursing Practice

Alistair Farley

Lecturer in Nursing, School of Nursing and Midwifery, University of Dundee, Dundee, UK

Ella McLafferty

Senior Lecturer in Nursing, School of Nursing and Midwifery, University of Dundee, Dundee, UK

Charles Hendry

Senior Lecturer in Nursing, School of Nursing and Midwifery, University of Dundee, Dundee, UK

WILEY-BLACKWELL

A John Wiley & Sons, Ltd., Publication

This edition first published 2011
© 2011 Alistair Farley, Ella McLafferty and Charles Hendry

Blackwell Publishing was acquired by John Wiley & Sons in February 2007. Blackwell's publishing programme has been merged with Wiley's global Scientific, Technical, and Medical business to form Wiley-Blackwell.

Registered office
John Wiley & Sons Ltd, The Atrium, Southern Gate, Chichester, West Sussex, PO19 8SQ, United Kingdom

Editorial offices
9600 Garsington Road, Oxford, OX4 2DQ, United Kingdom
The Atrium, Southern Gate, Chichester, West Sussex, PO19 8SQ, UK
2121 State Avenue, Ames, Iowa 50014-8300, USA

For details of our global editorial offices, for customer services and for information about how to apply for permission to reuse the copyright material in this book please see our website at www.wiley.com/wiley-blackwell.

Library of Congress Cataloging-in-Publication Data

Farley, Alistair.
    The physiological effects of ageing : implications for nursing practice /
Alistair Farley, Ella McLafferty, Charles Hendry.
        p. ; cm.
    Includes bibliographical references and index.
    ISBN 978-1-4051-8073-3 (pbk. : alk. paper)   1.   Geriatric nursing. 2.
Aging—Physiological aspects.   I. McLafferty, Ella. II. Hendry, Charles. III.
Title.
    [DNLM: 1.   Aging—physiology. 2.   Geriatric Assessment. 3.   Geriatric
Nursing—methods. 4.   Nursing Assessment.   WT 104]
    RC954.F367   2011
    618.97'0231—dc22

                                                                              2010041318

A catalogue record for this book is available from the British Library.

Set in 10/12.5 pt Times by MPS Limited, a Macmillan Company, Chennai, India
Printed and bound in Malaysia by Vivar Printing Sdn Bhd

1   2011

Contents

Author profiles

Alistair Farley

MSc in Nursing, BSc (Nursing), Dip Ed, Dip N (CT), RGN, RMN

Lecturer in Nursing, School of Nursing and Midwifery, University of Dundee, 11 Airlie Place, Dundee DD1 4HJ, UK

Alistair Farley has a background in trauma and orthopaedic nursing. He became a clinical nurse teacher in 1986 before qualifying as a lecturer in nursing in 1992. As a staff nurse in orthopaedics and a charge nurse in trauma, his nursing interests were focused on the acute management of patients. However, as many of the patients in an orthopaedic/trauma setting are older adults, he gradually developed an interest in this field of nursing. His experience and knowledge of older adults was further developed through his studies for his BSc and MSc in Nursing.

Ella McLafferty

PhD, BSc (Hons), Dip Ed, Dip N (CT), RGN, RM

Senior Lecturer in Nursing, School of Nursing and Midwifery, University of Dundee, 11 Airlie Place, Dundee DD1 4HJ, UK

Dr Ella McLafferty's main interest is older people nursing, although her background was originally in general nursing within surgical settings. Interest in older people's issues came about through working as a clinical teacher in a hospital that specialised in older people nursing. Through her BSc and her PhD, she has developed her knowledge in this field. She has had the opportunity to develop older adult nursing within nurse education.

Charles Hendry

PhD, BA (Hons), Dip Ed, Dip N (CT), RGN, RMN

Senior Lecturer in Nursing, School of Nursing and Midwifery, University of Dundee, 11 Airlie Place, Dundee DD1 4HJ, UK

Dr Charles Hendry has a background in Acute and Critical Care Nursing. As a clinician, educator and researcher, he knows the value of having the right information to provide focused and meaningful patient care. He has always believed in the importance of evidence-informed nursing practice and despite its many challenges would still recommend nursing as a career. Every day is different and it is a career in which you can make a real difference to people and their families.

Preface

It is our intention that this book will serve as a comprehensive resource for student nurses and qualified nurses who in the course of their work come into contact with older people. This book will also be of use to allied health professionals who want to develop their knowledge and understanding of the ageing process.

The aim of the book is to encourage all practitioners who work with older people to apply their knowledge of the ageing process to their practice and in doing so, enhance care delivery.

This book emphasises the normal ageing changes before considering possible effects of ageing on body systems, using as its framework Roper, Logan and Tierney's activities of living. Although problems associated with ageing are identified, nursing assessment and interventions are considered which can help reduce the impact these changes have on a person's functional ability.

Alistair Farley
Ella McLafferty
Charles Hendry

Chapter 1

Growing Older

Introduction

It is expected that the global population of older people will reach 20% of the total population by the year 2050, but this figure will be reached by 2020 in the United Kingdom (The House of Lords Science & Technology Committee, 2005). The number of older people will continue to increase over the next 15 years and beyond. The number of people in England aged over 90 is set to double between 1995 and 2025 (Department of Health (DH), 2001). The projection for Scotland is that by the year 2030 there will be more people in Scotland who are of retirement age than there will be children. The biggest growth is expected to be among the oldest old; in other words, the number of people aged over 80 is expected to double by the year 2030.

People over the age of 65 constitute the largest patient population in and out of hospital. More than 66% of patients who occupy acute care beds are over 65 years of age (DH, 2001). In 1998/99, the National Health Service (NHS) spent approximately 40% of its budget on those aged over 65 whilst social services spent nearly 50% on the same group (DH, 2001). Older people are traditionally admitted to hospital more frequently and for longer periods of time than younger people (Standing Nursing and Midwifery Advisory Committee (SNMAC), 2001). The DH (2001, p. 6) states that 'older people often require more intense, more skilled and more specialised nursing than younger adults'. Therefore, nursing older people requires well-prepared nurses to identify and manage their needs whether in hospital or at home.

The reality for most ageing people is that they have relatively good health, activity and independence (Feldman, 1999), with the ageing process being perceived not as something to be glorified but neither to be irrationally feared. That people are living longer is something to celebrate, reflecting the real achievements of organisations like the NHS, social services and the voluntary sector (DH, 2001). The DH goes on to state that older people should no longer be seen as a burden on society as they have vital resources of wisdom, experience and talent.

However, when older people are admitted to acute care settings they and their carers are the least satisfied with the care they receive when they are acutely ill (DH, 2001).

The Physiological Effects of Ageing: Implications for Nursing Practice, First Edition
© Alistair Farley, Ella McLafferty and Charles Hendry
Published 2011 by Blackwell Publishing Ltd

Hospital admission itself can dramatically reduce the physical and psychological ability of an older person to self-care (Clark, 1998). A combination of actions such as infantilisation (treating older adults like children), fostered dependency, not listening or offering choices can all contribute to the objectification of an older person in care (Nay, 1998). Hancock et al. (2003) identified that hospitalisation for an older person is associated with a decline in health and increased dependency. This decline in health and associated loss of independence may prevent the older adult from being discharged home, making it more likely that they will have to be transferred into long-term care. In their study, Hancock et al. (2003) identified that nurses felt that they did not have enough time to provide all aspects of care to hospitalised older adults. This situation can easily be rectified by ensuring that more staff are available to care for the older population.

Nurse education specifically in the care of older people is vital if they are to receive the care they require. Older patients tend to present as more acutely unwell than younger patients and are more likely to be dependent on nurses because of co-morbidities. There is also huge pressure to discharge patients from hospital as early as possible in their pathway. However, this does not take into account the effects of the ageing process combined with the effects of stressors on the speed of recovery. Edwards et al. (2008) have identified that nursing students need to be prepared specifically to care for older people. It is imperative that nursing students have a thorough grounding in the care of older people as they will meet older people in most clinical settings in the hospital and in the community.

Drivers in the care of older adults

A number of drivers have been published to improve the care delivered to older people. One of the most influential drivers has been the National Service Framework for Older People published by the DH in 2001. This is a comprehensive strategy to enable the delivery of fair, high-quality, integrated health and social care services for older people.

The aim of this strategy is to support independence and promote good health for older people, and to try and ensure that older people and their carers are treated with respect, dignity and fairness.

The strategy rightly identifies that older people live for many years into retirement as fit and healthy individuals. Old age is described as beginning at 60 for women and 65 for men. Although entitlement to the state pension is in the process of being equalised so that by the year 2020 women will be entitled to the pension if they are 65 years old. However, the goals of health and social care policy are to promote and extend healthy and active life and to compress morbidity.

There are four main themes in the National Service Framework (NSF) (DH, 2001):

- Respecting the individual
- Intermediate care
- Promoting evidence-based specialist care
- Promoting an active and healthy life.

The Scottish Executive in 2005 produced the document Building a Health Service Fit for the Future, which puts forward a strategy to manage the shifting patterns of disease in an ageing population in order to take account of the number of older people with multiple conditions, especially long-term conditions and for those with complex needs.

They identify the need to move from a reactive to a proactive approach and reduce the risks of some health problems or to manage them appropriately and that is the purpose of this book, to give nursing students the knowledge and the tools to manage older people's issues in order to reduce or minimise their problems.

Documents producing specific protocols and guidelines that are relevant to the care of older people have also been published. NICE Guidelines giving best practice for falls in older people were produced in 2004 (CG 21) while guidelines to promote older people's mental well-being have been produced in 2008 (PH 16).

The National Health Service Quality Improvement Service (NHSQIS) produce standard statements on a variety of nursing issues. The role of the NHSQIS is to lead the use of knowledge to promote improvement in the quality of health care for people in Scotland. They have produced standard statements for Nutrition in Older People in 2002 and Oral Health in Older People in 2005 among many others.

Activities of living

The framework for this book is based on the model of nursing originally described by Roper et al., in the publication *The Elements of Nursing* in 1980. This model for nursing based on a model of living has been used widely in clinical practice areas to guide the management of nursing care and has been used in many Schools of Nursing and Midwifery to aid students in the linking of nursing theory to nursing practice (Roper et al., 2000). Curricula have also been based around this particular model. The aim of the model is to identify the management of a patient by identifying patients' abilities to carry out the activities of living. The model is divided into two parts. Part 1 is the model of living and part 2 is the model of nursing. The model of living consists of five main components: activities of living, lifespan, dependence/ independence, factors influencing the activities of living and individuality in living. There are 12 activities of living, and these are the activities that we carry out in order to live from day to day. The activities, although considered separately, do overlap. The lifespan is a continuum from birth to death. The dependence–independence continuum acknowledges that a person, depending on where they are in their lifespan, may not be able to be fully independent through stages of life or through illness. This continuum is inextricably linked to the activities of living. There are five factors that influence the activities of living and they include:

- Biological factors
- Psychological factors
- Sociocultural factors
- Environmental factors
- Politico-economic factors.

This book is based around old age in the lifespan. We emphasise the importance of maintaining and promoting independence in older people, and we concentrate on the biological factors associated with the ageing process. Not all of the activities of living have been utilised. As has already been stated, this is a book about the physiological aspects of ageing and not all of the activities are relevant for this purpose. This book has been written around the following activities of living:

- Maintaining a safe environment
- Communicating
- Breathing
- Eating and drinking
- Eliminating
- Controlling body temperature
- Mobilising
- Expressing sexuality
- Sleeping.

The activities that have not been included within the book are:

- Personal cleansing and dressing
- Working and playing
- Dying.

The rationale for excluding these three activities are that the physiological effects of ageing for personal cleansing and dressing are included in other chapters such as mobilising and changes associated with the skin as well as oral health which is included in the activity of eating and drinking. There are no physiological effects associated with working and playing, although physiological changes in other activities may influence the ability to carry out activities associated with living and working. The process of dying has been excluded as it is similar for many people no matter their age, and the issues associated with dying are also similar.

Overall aims

This book should support the theoretical component of the undergraduate nursing curriculum relating to nursing older people. Undergraduate programmes in the United Kingdom provide an academic and professional qualification through integrated study of theory and supervised nursing practice in NHS and independent clinical settings. The curriculum should conform in the main to recommendations by the Nursing and Midwifery Advisory Committee (2001) regarding the achievement of fundamental skills required by Registered Nurses to meet the needs of older people. Gerontological education plays an important role in countering ageism; therefore, greater attention is required in relation to gerontological nursing within curricula, as how information presented can influence learning (Happell and Brooker, 2001).

The aim of this book is to describe the normal physiological effects of ageing. Every organism ages, and humans are no different. This book emphasises that the ageing process is normal and is not directly responsible for disease. However, some diseases and problems become more prevalent as we grow older and some disorders can be minimised or prevented. These issues will be addressed in this book. We need to appreciate that the ageing body is efficient and effective in that there is spare capacity associated with most systems of the body that allow our body to cope with the loss of cells as we age and feel little effect from these losses. There are also efficient and effective compensatory mechanisms used by a number of the body systems ensuring that the functioning of the whole person continues often with no apparent (or perhaps minimal) reduction in ability.

Problems that are commonly found among older people are also considered including their assessment and management. It is not the purpose of this book to provide a comprehensive text on the disorders of ageing, but rather by selecting some common health problems of older adults, the reader will be able to make strong links between anatomy and physiology and the changes that occur in older adults.

This book is written with the intention of providing nurses and other health-care professionals with a comprehensive text relating to the ageing process. From the outset, we wish to make it clear that in this book we will focus primarily on the physiological impact of growing older; however, this is not to minimise the significance of the psychological, social and spiritual elements of human being. Lecturers too will find it useful as we believe that it is the only text of its kind that provides a comprehensive account of the physiological effects of ageing.

If there is one thing that we all have in common it is the fact that each and everyday we are all getting older. However, it is important to state at the outset that ageing is a normal process and does not necessarily lead to disease and disability. Ageing is inevitable and irreversible. However, it is acknowledged that with advancing age comes a decline in functional ability of each organ and system (Herbert, 1992). Nevertheless, individuals do not age at the same pace and within each individual, systems and organs age at different rates. Experience also tells us that the consequences of ageing vary greatly between individuals.

Lifestyle, environment and family history all play a part in how we age; however, how we each experience growing older is in part determined by our own philosophies and outlook on life. The following chapters will, we hope, prepare the health-care professionals of tomorrow to provide advice and care for older adults which will allow them to derive maximum benefit from their 'golden years'.

References

Clark, J. 1998. Clinical Standards Advisory Group: Community Health Care for Elderly People. The Stationery Office, London.

Department of Health. 2001. The National Service Framework for Older People. The Stationery Office, London.

Edwards, H., Nash, R., Sacre, S., Courtney, M. and Abbey, J. 2008. Development of a virtual learning environment to enhance undergraduate nursing students' effectiveness and interest in working with older people. Nurse Education Today 28(6), 672–679.

Feldman, S. 1999. Please don't call me 'dear': older women's narratives of health care. Nursing Inquiry 6(4), 269–276.

Hancock, K., Chang, E., Chenoweth, L., Clarke, M., Carroll, A. and Jeon, Y.H. 2003. Nursing needs of acutely ill older people. Journal of Advanced Nursing 44(5), 507–516.

Happell, B. and Brooker, J. 2001. Who will look after my grandmother? Attitudes of student nurses toward the care of older adults. Journal of Gerontological Nursing 27(12), 12–17.

Herbert, R. 1992. The normal aging process reviewed. International Nursing Review 39(3), 93–96.

House of Lords' Science & Technology Committee. 2005. Ageing: Scientific Aspects, Vol. 1: Report. The Stationery Office, London.

National Health Service Quality Improvement Scotland. 2002. Nutrition in Older People. NHSQIS, Edinburgh.

National Health Service Quality Improvement Scotland. 2005. Oral Health in Older People. NHSQIS, Edinburgh.

Nay, R. 1998. Contradictions between perceptions and practices of caring in long-term care of the elderly. Journal of Clinical Nursing 7(5), 401–408.

NICE. 2004. Best Practice for Falls in Older People. CG21. NICE, London.

NICE. 2008. Guidelines to Promote Older People's Mental Wellbeing. PH16. NICE, London.

Nursing and Midwifery Advisory Committee. 2001. Caring for Older People: A Nursing Priority. Department of Health, London.

Roper, N., Logan, W. and Tierney, A. 2000. The Roper, Logan and Tierney Model of Nursing. Churchill Livingstone, Edinburgh.

Scottish Executive. 2005. Building a Health Service Fit for the Future. Scottish Executive, Edinburgh.

Chapter 2

Theories of Ageing

Aims

After reading this chapter you will be able to discuss the current theories of biological ageing and consider how these may account for the physiological changes seen in the older adult.

Learning Outcomes

After completion of this chapter you will be able to:

- Outline the principal biological theories of ageing
- Discuss how ageing may impact upon the older adult's physiological functioning
- Examine how ageing may effect homeostasis
- Reflect upon how ageing impacts upon the older adult's recovery from illness.

Introduction

We will begin this chapter with an examination of a number of current theories that propose a mechanism for the phenomenon of ageing. We will then go on to discuss the effects of ageing on homeostasis and body function.

Ageing theories

Scientists agree that there would appear to be no single mechanism of ageing (Kirkwood, 2003). Rather, it is suggested that there are multiple mechanisms which over time result in a deterioration in general cellular function and a less vigorous response to internal and

The Physiological Effects of Ageing: Implications for Nursing Practice, First Edition
© Alistair Farley, Ella McLafferty and Charles Hendry
Published 2011 by Blackwell Publishing Ltd

external stressors. Most theories agree that the cumulative cellular damage associated with ageing is a consequence of the body's failure to adequately repair this damage. These mechanisms, as stated earlier, are considered to be metabolically harmful. They include mutations in DNA, defective mitochondria, oxidative damage over time by the presence of free radicals and a build-up of atypical proteins. It can be seen, therefore, that ageing is a result of a gradual amassing of faults in the cells and tissues within the body (Kirkwood, 2003), changes which contribute to an increased risk of chronic disease and death.

We will now go on to consider a number of different theories of ageing.

Error theory

Increases in somatic mutations associated with the ageing process can result in alterations in the genetic sequences within DNA (Montague et al., 2005). By somatic we mean the non-sex cells within the body. Error theory or error catastrophe theory suggests that these changes in DNA are passed onto the next generation of cells (Ricklefs and Finch, 1995). These new cells, containing altered DNA, will produce proteins which are different from the original ones, that is, deviant proteins. The next generation of cells will also contain this deviation, and this will continue until eventually the cells being produced are significantly different from the original parent cell. Error theory suggests that this leads to a diminished functional ability of the resulting cell line. Over time tissues, organs and systems demonstrate a reduction in reserve capacity. Initially, the individual may only notice this reduction in function with exertion or strenuous activity, but as more functionality is lost, this may become increasingly evident with less activity or even at rest.

Free radical theory

The free radical theory of ageing was first discussed by Harman in 1956. Free radicals are molecules with one or more unpaired electrons in their outer orbits. These atoms are therefore very unstable and try to initiate rapid chemical reactions in an attempt to form more stable molecules. During this process, free radicals attack and modify other molecules (Ricklefs and Finch, 1995). Free radicals are produced normally within the body as a by-product of cell metabolism. Although there are many different types of free radicals, it would appear that oxygen radicals are the most pathological to the human body (Woodrow, 2002). In a very real sense, whilst we need oxygen to live, oxygen is also a poison. Free radicals are therefore toxic compounds produced when oxygen is metabolised.

Free radicals are normally eliminated within the body by enzymes found in peroxisomes and cytosol (Tortora, 2005). However, an accumulation of free radicals can cause oxidative damage to cellular structures including cell proteins, cell membranes and nucleic acids. Over time this damage leads to cell mutation and senescence (Amella, 2004). Oxidative stress is strongly linked to the ageing process, and a major target for oxidative damage is DNA (House of Lords Science and Technology Committee, 2005).

Accumulation of damage by the recurrent effects of free radicals within the body has been linked to the development of several chronic diseases, including cardiovascular disease, respiratory disease, cancers and dementia (Khaw, 1997), which may not necessarily be associated with ageing. A very visible demonstration of damage caused by the presence of free radicals is 'age spots', or Lentigo, which are pigmented areas of skin caused by deposition of lipofuscin, a by-product of free radical activity. Lipofuscin causes deprivation of oxygen and nutrients to healthy tissue eventually leading to its death (Meiner and Lueckenotte, 2006).

It is known that exposure to a number of factors can increase the production of free radicals within the body and hence also increase the damage associated with their presence. These factors include:

- Cigarette smoke
- Infection
- Toxins
- A diet high in saturated fats.

The production of free radicals is also appreciably increased following exposure to ionising radiation such as prolonged and excessive exposure to the sun or accumulative exposure to X-rays (Nowak and Handford, 1996).

Seeley et al. (2003) and Meiner and Lueckenotte (2006) suggest that antioxidants (free radical foragers) such as vitamin C, beta-carotene, selenium and vitamin E may alleviate the damage caused by free radicals. Antioxidants prevent oxidation (and subsequent damage) of cell components by donating an electron to the outer orbit of the free radicals and in this way make them more stable (Seeley et al., 2003).

Activity

Identify foods that are good sources of vitamin C, beta-carotene, selenium and vitamin E.

Immune theory

There is a decline in immunocompetence in the older adult. The immune theory of ageing proposes that as the immune system deteriorates over time, the resulting decline in function contributes to the development of cancers, opportunistic infections and other immune associated diseases. Whilst T and B lymphocyte function declines, macrophage activity can actually increase contributing to sustained inflammation and swelling (Ricklefs and Finch, 1995). Matteson (1997) also suggests that autoantibodies accumulate in the body with advancing age, which then direct the immune system to attack 'self' cells, that is, the body's own cells. It is suggested that this may be due to the effects of age-related changes in cells. Cells reach a point where they are no longer recognised as 'self' and are therefore viewed as foreign and targeted by the immune system.

Montague et al. (2005) suggest that, in addition, alterations in amino acids result in changes to protein synthesis. These altered proteins can then be viewed as 'non-self' triggering an immune response.

The overall efficiency and effectiveness of our immune system can be enhanced by taking zinc, selenium, vitamin A and riboflavin and by participating in exercise. However, experimental studies have shown that chronic nicotine exposure has an effect on the animal immune systems and may contribute to nicotine/cigarette smoke-induced immuno-suppression (Geng et al., 1995, 1996). Arcavi and Benowitz (2004) suggest that smoking not only increases the risk of infections due to structural changes in the respiratory tract, but also results in a decrease in immune response, thereby putting smokers at greater risk of opportunistic infections.

Activity

Identify your local 'stop smoking' resources. These may be a health promotion professional, a drop-in clinic, self-help groups, health advice leaflets, etc. Using these local resources, explore the strategies that you may employ to assist an older person give up smoking.

Programmed theory of ageing: changes in cell replication

Each cell in the body has its origin in an original fertilised ovum. All subsequent generations of cells result from a parent cell dividing and producing daughter cells. Each daughter cell then divides in its turn and so on throughout life. During embryonic development cells must also differentiate into different cell types.

The programmed theory of ageing suggests that cells have a finite, or limited, number of times that they can divide, or replicate. When they reach this limit, they become unable to continue replication. The cell recognises this limit and triggers a cell death sequence known as apoptosis. As more and more cells reach this stage, functional ability declines and obvious signs of ageing appear.

Telomeres are sections of DNA that protect the ends of chromosomes from decay and from sticking to one another.

 Revision Point

If you are unsure of the structure of DNA and chromosomes, you might find it helpful to review this in your preferred textbook.

However, with each subsequent cell division the telomeres shorten. After many cycles of cell division, the telomeres are significantly reduced in size and no longer able to protect the chromosome. In the absence of this protective 'cap', the chromosomes themselves 'fray' and deteriorate over time, leading to a breakdown in the organism's genetic material. This disruption in the chromosome prevents cells from replicating and can lead to cellular damage, cell death or cancer (Amella, 2004).

Telomerase is an enzyme found in abundance in cancerous cells but not in non-cancerous cells (Mauk, 2006; Meiner and Lueckenotte, 2006). This enzyme prevents the shortening of telomeres after cell division and therefore prevents the cell from dying after a finite number of divisions where the telomeres would have been used up (Lueckenotte,

Table 2.1   Theories of ageing (adapted from Farley et al. (2006), with permission from the RCN).

Theories	Description
Error theory	Alteration in the sequencing of genes in DNA. Error theory suggests that this leads to decreased functional ability of the cell.
Free radical theory	Free radicals are toxic compounds leading to oxidative stress that damages DNA. Accumulation of damage by the recurrent effects of free radicals within the body has been linked to the development of several chronic diseases.
Immune theory	Decline in immune system functioning where age-related changes in cells may result in them no longer being recognised as 'self' and therefore seen as foreign and targeted by the immune system. Or an increase in autoimmune responses where altered proteins are viewed as 'non-self' triggering an immune response.
Programmed theory of ageing: changes in cell replication	Loss of telomeres disrupts cell replication. This disruption in the chromosome prevents cells from replicating and can lead to cellular damage, cellular death or cancer.
Neuroendocrine theory	The secretion of a range of hormones from the neuroendocrine system begins to fail with age. These changes result in an increase in disease in a number of body systems and organs.

2000). Cancerous cells are not governed by the same rules as non-cancerous cells (Siegel, 2008) and as such they maintain their telomeres and therefore can continue to divide indefinitely. This may account for the increasing incidence of cancers seen in older adults. It also opens up the possibility of treatments aimed at blocking the action of telomerase, thus preventing cancer cells from multiplying.

Neuroendocrine theory

We know that the nervous and endocrine systems play a key role in regulating normal growth, repair and development. It is postulated that as we age the regulatory pathways and the secretion of a range of hormones from the neuroendocrine system begin to fail. Notably, these include the hormones oestrogen, growth hormone and melatonin (Mauk, 2006). Plasma cortisol levels have also been shown to increase as a result of increased activation of the hypothalamus–pituitary–adrenal axis. The net effect of these changes is an increase in disease in a number of body systems and organs.

See Table 2.1 for a brief description of these ageing theories.

Effects of ageing on homeostasis and body function

Homeostasis is the maintenance of a constant internal environment which is necessary for effective physiological activity. Homeostasis involves a complex series of physiological and biochemical changes and responses. Nearly all organs and systems are involved in this process (Redfern and Ross, 2001). Whilst homeostasis is maintained in older adults, functional ability will decline over time. This decline may not be obvious or uniform and may not necessarily interfere with a person's social functioning. However, a combination of stressors (internal or external) and ageing changes can have a deleterious effect on homeostasis. Such stressors can include illness, trauma, exposure to extreme environmental temperatures and strenuous exercise. These stressors may impact negatively on homeostasis in the older adult as although they have reserve capacity in organ systems, this capacity is reduced to the point where it cannot match the demands made by these stressors. In other words, systems which may normally function well most of the time can be overwhelmed by illness, trauma, infection and other stressors. When this occurs, the individual is no longer in homeostasis and problems ensue. When such a state is reached, it takes longer for the older adult to recover and return to the pre-stressor condition.

Reserve capacity is the spare capacity that systems have which ordinarily are not used but will be available if needed. A person uses their reserve capacity when there are increased health demands made on the body. Reduction in reserve capacity is an important consideration in frailty. Borz (2002) states that all organ systems of the body show evidence of redundant structure and function, stating that most systems have as much as a 70% margin of loss before signs of failure become apparent. Consequently, 30% of normal functioning is adequate for most needs. However, the reserve capacity becomes significant during episodes of stress, injury or illness, and as stated earlier, in older adults this reserve capacity is diminished, making it more likely that they succumb to illness.

Summary

Contrary to the impression that we often have of ageing, growing older is not synonymous with disease and infirmity. Regardless of which theory or theories of ageing proves to be correct, older adults can, for the most part, continue to lead a full and active life and maintain their usual daily activities.

However, the loss of 'spare capacity' in organs and systems may be significant when the older adult becomes unwell. Recovery from illness is slower in older adults and health-care professionals need to plan accordingly.

It is also important to acknowledge that there is a psychological, social and spiritual as well as physiological dimension to growing older. It is not our intention in this text to examine these elements of ageing; however, the reader is directed to further reading if they wish to pursue this further.

For health-care professionals, knowledge of current theories of ageing should help them to advise adults about particular risks or compounding factors such as obesity or smoking. In this way, they can assist the ageing adult to maintain an optimum level of health for as long as possible and help them to adapt their activities of living when and if required.

References and further reading

Amella, E.J. 2004. Presentation of illness in older adults. American Journal of Nursing 104(10), 40–51.

Arcavi, L. and Benowitz, N.L. 2004. Cigarette smoking and infection. Archives of Internal Medicine 164(20), 2206–2216.

Borz, W.M., II. 2002. A conceptual framework of frailty: a review. The Journals of Gerontology Series A: Biological Sciences and Medical Sciences 57(5), 283–288.

Farley, A.H., McLafferty, E. and Hendry, C. 2006. The physiological effects of ageing on the activities of living. Nursing Standard 20(45), 46–52.

Geng, Y., Savage, S.M., Johnson, L.J., Seagrave, J. and Sopori, M.L. 1995. Effects of nicotine on the immune response. I. Chronic exposure to nicotine impairs antigen receptor-mediated signal transduction in lymphocytes. Toxicology and Applied Pharmacology 135(2), 268–278.

Geng, Y., Savage, S.M., Razani-Boroujerdi, S. and Sopori, M.L. 1996. Effects of nicotine on the immune response. II. Chronic nicotine treatment induces T cell anergy. Journal of Immunology 156(7), 2384–2390.

Harman, D. 1956. Aging: a theory based on the free radical and radiation chemistry. Journal of Gerontology 11(3), 298–300.

House of Lords Science and Technology Committee. 2005. Scientific Aspects of Ageing. The Stationary Office, London.

Khaw, K. 1997. Healthy aging. British Medical Journal 315(7115), 1090–1096.

Kirkwood, T.B. 2003. The most pressing problem of our age. British Medical Journal 326(7402), 1297–1299.

Lueckenotte, A.G. 2000. Gerontologic Nursing. 2nd ed. Mosby, St. Louis, MO.

Matteson, M.A. 1997. Biological theories of ageing. In Matteson, M.A., McConnell, E.S. and Linton, A.D. (Eds). Gerontological Nursing: Concepts and Practice. 2nd ed. Saunders, Philadelphia, PA, pp. 159–171.

Mauk, K.L. 2006. Gerontological Nursing: Competencies for Care. Jones and Bartlett Publishers, Sudbury, MA.

Meiner, S.E. and Lueckenotte, A.G. 2006. Gerontologic Nursing. 3rd ed. Mosby Elsevier, St. Louis, MO.

Montague, S., Watson, R. and Herbert, R. 2005. Physiology for Nursing Practice. 3rd ed. Elsevier, Edinburgh.

Nowak, T.J. and Handford, A.G. 1996. Essentials of Pathophysiology. WC Brown Publishers, Dubuque, IA.

Redfern, S.J. and Ross, F.M. 2001. Nursing Older People. 3rd ed. Churchill Livingstone, Edinburgh.

Ricklefs, R.E. and Finch, C.E. 1995. Aging: A Natural History. Scientific American Library, New York, NY.

Seeley, R.R., Stephens, T.D. and Tate, P. 2003. Anatomy and Physiology. 6th ed. McGraw Hill, London.

Siegel, L.J. 2008. Are telomeres the key to aging and cancer. http://learn.genetics.utah.edu/content/begin/traits/telomeres/index.html. Last accessed 4th May 2009.

Tortora, G. 2005. Principals of Human Anatomy. 10th ed. Wiley, Hoboken, NJ.

Woodrow, P. 2002. Ageing: Issues for Physical, Psychological and Social Health. Whurr, London.

Chapter 3

Maintaining a Safe Environment

Aims

After reading this chapter you will be able to discuss how the immune system protects the body from harm and how deficits in this system may impair the health of older adults.

Learning Outcomes

After completion of this chapter you will be able to:

- Describe the normal structure and function of the immune system
- Conduct a comprehensive patient assessment of the above systems using appropriate tools
- Detail the changes in the above system that are associated with ageing
- Discuss the presentation and management of HIV/AIDS as it occurs in older adults.

Introduction

This chapter will start with an overview of the normal anatomy and physiology of the immune system and how this works to protect the person from harm. We will consider the acute inflammatory response as this is a fundamental protective response of the immune system. We shall then go on to look briefly at wound healing.

Changes in how the older adult's immune system responds to challenges will be considered before we look at the issue of HIV/AIDS and older people.

The Physiological Effects of Ageing: Implications for Nursing Practice, First Edition
© Alistair Farley, Ella McLafferty and Charles Hendry
Published 2011 by Blackwell Publishing Ltd

Immune system

The immune system is the body's defence system. This protection is provided by two complementary responses, namely the innate or non-specific immune response and the adaptive or specific immune response.

The innate immune responses occur in a number of different ways.

Physical/mechanical and chemical barriers

The major physical and chemical barriers to infection are the skin and mucous membranes that line the gastrointestinal (GI), respiratory and genital tracts.

Intact skin is the major barrier to the entry of organisms to the body. If the skin is damaged in any way this protective barrier can be compromised. In addition, the slightly acidic pH of the skin as a result of sweat and sebaceous gland secretions inhibits certain bacterial growth. The presence of commensal bacteria (living on or within another organism without causing harm to the host) can also be deemed protective as access to the site may be prevented or key nutrients may be used up, thereby preventing colonisation by potentially harmful bacteria.

The mucous membranes of the respiratory system secrete a protective layer of mucus which can trap potentially harmful material, and the mechanical movement of the respiratory cilia aided by the coughing and sneezing reflexes also help prevent the entry of pathogenic organisms to the lower respiratory tract.

The presence of hydrochloric acid in the stomach helps create an environment where the acidity helps protect against microbial survival. The antibacterial enzyme lysozyme that is present in breast milk, tears, nasal secretions and saliva also protects against harmful bacteria. The continual flow of tears and saliva wash away debris and bacteria and thereby help to protect the eyes and mouth from being colonised by potentially harmful microorganisms. The simple action of passing urine can also be deemed as protective, as the action of emptying the bladder can 'flush' away microorganisms from the bladder or urethra.

Phagocytosis

Phagocytosis is a process whereby non-self or foreign substances are recognised as such and consumed by a group of white blood cells known as leucocytes. The two types largely responsible for phagocytosis are neutrophils and macrophages.

Before adhering to and digesting foreign material, it must first be recognised as non-self tissue, that is, we must recognise it as foreign material. Specialised proteins or receptors on white blood cells attach themselves to the cell wall of the bacteria. When this occurs, the area where the attachment has taken place acts as a chemical 'tag' or label identifying the bacteria as non-self tissue and as such it becomes a target for phagocytosis.

Once this contact has been made, the white blood cell (phagocytic) engulfs the organism by throwing extensions of its plasma membrane and cytoplasm (pseudopodia) around it until the phagocytic cell completely covers the organism. The organism is then brought into the cytoplasm of the phagocytic cell where it fuses (joins) with organelles called lysosomes. These lysosomes contain digestive enzymes which then break down the ingested organism.

Acute inflammatory response

The inflammatory response is initiated in response to any infection or assault. The reaction leads to redness, heat, swelling, pain/discomfort and impaired function of the affected part. Damaged tissues release many chemical transmitters including histamine. The release of these chemical transmitters promotes vasodilation (resulting in heat and redness of the surrounding area) and increased capillary permeability (which increases the amount of fluid entering the interstitial space, thereby producing oedema and the sensation of pain).

The injured area is isolated from the surrounding healthy tissue as fibrinogen clots form around the injured site. This restricts the area of damage and reduces the spread of potentially harmful microorganisms. Leucocytes are attracted to the area of damage by the process of chemotaxis and they begin the process of phagocytosis. Macrophages arrive later and continue with the process of phagocytosis. Lymphatic vessels surrounding the area remove excess fluid, cell debris and dead microorganisms.

Other non-specific responses include the use of natural killer (NK) cells which are mainly directed at virus-infected cells. The NK cells bind to virus particles on the surface of infected cells and secrete a substance known as perforin, a pore-forming protein. Release of perforin damages the cell membrane resulting in cellular death which prevents the virus from replicating.

Interferons are a group of proteins produced by lymphocytes and macrophages when invaded by virus. The release of interferons enhances the activity of surrounding NK cells, macrophages and cells of the specific immune response. These actions speed up removal of the invading microorganism. The presence of interferons also induces the resistance of host cells to viral infection.

Complement activity is another non-specific response to the presence of microorganisms. The activation of the complement cascade enhances or complements the body's many defensive actions. Complement activity involves the action of a group of proteins found in the blood which when stimulated form what is known as the complement cascade, the end product being a protein called membrane attack complex. The resulting membrane attack complex results in the destruction of the microorganism's cell membrane and thereby its death.

One feature of all of the components of the innate immune response is that they do not improve over time or upon repeated exposure to potentially harmful microorganisms.

However, the response of the adaptive (specific) immune response does improve upon subsequent exposure to the stimulus of a particular trigger and, once stimulated, the adaptive immune response 'remembers' the encounter with specific triggers and the reaction is much more vigorous in second and subsequent exposures.

An antigen is any substance capable of provoking an immune response and is normally foreign to the organism. Antibodies are highly specific proteins produced by B cells in response to the presence of an antigen.

Cells of the adaptive immune response are known as B cells (B lymphocytes) and T cells (T lymphocytes). B cells are particularly effective in destroying bacteria and inactivating their toxins (Tortora, 2005). They work mainly through the production of specific proteins known as antibodies. Following their production, antibodies are released into the general circulation where they find and bind onto specific receptor sites on the invading agent.

T cells are active against damaged and infected body cells. There are three subsets of T cells. Cytotoxic T cells kill by using toxic and pore-forming chemicals. However, unlike NK cells, they must be bound to antigen and receive additional signals from another type of T cell, the helper T cell. Helper T cells regulate the overall immune response. They 'switch on' the immune response, increase the rate and intensity of the response, they boost the effectiveness of the innate response and prolong the inflammatory reaction. These effects are achieved through the release of chemical known as lymphokines. When the response is no longer required, they also activate suppressor T cells which then release their own lymphokines to dampen down the overall response.

After the successful removal of the offending organism, memory cells of both B and T lymphocytes remain. These help produce a rapid and violent response on the next encounter with the same offending organism/agent.

Typical immune response to the presence of pathogenic microorganisms

When an antigen enters the body, macrophages phagocytose these and present some of the molecules of antigen to the lymphocytes found in lymph nodes. Each B lymphocyte found in the lymph node has about 100 000 surface immunoglobulins (surface proteins) on its surface membrane which act as receptors for a specific antigen. When the macrophage presents the antigen to the appropriate receptor, they join together (bind). This binding together of antigen and receptor, plus activating signals from T cells, causes the appropriate B cell to proliferate – it enlarges and multiplies, giving rise to plasma cells and memory cells.

Plasma cells produce, and release, antibodies into the circulation. These antibodies have the same receptor for antigen as their parent B cell, that is, the antibodies produced are an exact and specific match for the original stimulating antigen. Their ability to act as receptor for antigen is the very same as their parent B cell. Once in circulation, released antibodies exert their effect in a number of ways:

- They bind to antigens, clumping them together, making them an easier target for phagocytosis.
- When bound to antigen, the antibody also acts as a chemical marker or opsonin, again leading to enhancement of phagocytosis.
- The act of binding, together with signals from T cells, triggers another defence response known as the complement cascade.
- The binding of antibody and antigen will also trigger an acute inflammatory reaction.

Relationship between innate (non-specific) and acquired (specific) immunity

The collaboration between innate and acquired immunity is extensive. Adaptive immunity relies upon innate immunity in that antigens must be prepared by cells such as macrophages before they can be presented to B and T cells. Helper T cells require an activating signal (lymphokine) secreted by macrophages. In addition, macrophages also secrete chemotactic factors that are responsible for attracting T and B cells to the area under attack.

Adaptive immunity regulates and enhances innate immunity in a number of ways, for example lymphokines secreted by helper T cells promote the proliferation, maturation and activation of all cells involved in innate immunity. Antibodies focus the mechanisms of innate immunity on to the targets to which they bind and promote phagocytosis by opsonisation of antigens and trigger the complement cascade.

Wound healing

The process of wound healing is a complex series of events that begins at the time of injury and can continue for months or even years. The phases involved in wound healing are inflammation, reconstruction, epithelialisation and maturation.

The inflammatory response begins almost immediately after injury and lasts for about 3 days. Initially, there is reflex vasoconstriction of damaged blood vessels which narrows the lumen and reduces blood loss. Thrombocytes join together to form a loose platelet plug which is stabilised by fibrin. Over time, a blood clot forms which prevents further blood loss from the damaged vessels.

Blood vessels which surround the damaged area vasodilate. This is due to the release of various chemicals from the injured tissue and basophils. The vasodilation of local blood vessels increases the flow of blood to and from the injured area. The chemical release, including histamine, also increases the permeability of the surrounding blood vessel walls. This allows fluid and cells, especially white blood cells, within the blood to leave the blood vessels and go to the area of damage. These responses to tissue damage/injury give rise to the cardinal signs of inflammation – redness, heat, swelling, pain and a change in function. Redness and heat are due to the increased flow of blood through the damaged area and do not necessarily indicate the presence of infection. Swelling and pain are due to fluid movement from blood vessels to the tissues causing pressure on nerve endings or irritation due to the presence of these chemicals. A change in function may be due to the combination of these factors. White blood cells that are attracted to the damaged area by chemotaxis identify non-self tissue and damaged self tissue and begin the process of removing these through the action of phagocytosis. Potentially harmful microorganisms are also identified and removed by phagocytosis. The white blood cells that are particularly active during this phase are leucocytes and macrophages.

During the reconstruction phase, the white blood cells identified above clear the area of all unwanted material and microorganisms. Fibroblasts are recruited to the area and begin to produce proteins such as collagen and elastin. Fibroblast activity results in new connective tissue being formed which is supplied with blood by the production of new blood vessels. In this way, oxygen and nutrients are brought to the new tissue and metabolic wastes are removed. The new tissue gradually strengthens as collagen fibres reorganise within the wound and produce what is known as granulation tissue. This tissue is delicate and care will be required when managing the wound, although it will strengthen in time.

The regrowth of epithelial cells over the surface of the wound is termed epithelialisation. Various cells including cells from sebaceous and sweat glands divide and migrate over the surface of the wound. If slough or necrotic tissue is present, they should be removed as their presence will reduce the rate of regrowth of epithelial cells.

The final phase of wound healing is maturation, where the collagen matrix becomes tighter and more organised. The number of fibroblasts also decreases. The vascularity of the wound decreases and the wound appears pale in colour. Tissue maturation continues over weeks and months and in some instances, where there is a large open wound, may take years. Despite the actions described earlier, the final tensile strength of a wound does not exceed 80% of the original tissue.

 Point for Practice

Using your knowledge of wound healing, identify strategies for promoting tissue repair in older adults.

Ageing changes in the immune system

The immune system reaches its functional peak around the period of puberty, after which it reduces its capacity over a person's lifespan by between 5% and 30% (Carter and Pottinger, 2001). Despite ageing changes, the immune system continues to maintain its defensive function even in very old adults. However, some, but not all, aspects of the immune system do decline with advancing age (Ginaldi and Sternberg, 2003). Therefore, it should not come as a surprise that very old people are more likely to die of infectious diseases including pneumonia, influenza and gastro-enteritis among others. This can be directly linked to the ageing changes in the immune system as it no longer protects to the same level when compared with younger people (Ginaldi and Sternberg, 2003). Not only are older people at greater risk of dying from infections, but they also respond differently to the presence of microorganisms. Infection can occur in older people on exposure to reduced number of microorganisms as compared with younger adults. Older people may also respond differently to infections when compared with younger people. Urinary tract infection (UTI) is a good example where a different response occurs in older adults who commonly present with signs of confusion prior to signs of pyrexia. Symptoms of infection may also be masked or mistaken for other diseases, or symptoms may appear less severe (Carter and Pottinger, 2001).

Other factors can impact on older people's ability to combat infection and they should also be considered. These include taking medications that can increase the risk of infection. Examples of these drugs include steroids and anti-inflammatory medications both of which reduce the inflammatory response. Older people are at risk from long-term conditions such as diabetes and chronic obstructive pulmonary disease (COPD) and their presence can also increase the likelihood of infection.

Changes in the immune system due to the ageing process are called immuno-senescence. There seems to be a significant reduction in the immune system's ability to respond efficiently and changes occur both in the innate elements of the immune system and the adaptive elements of the system (Linton, 2007). The changes in innate immunity presents as a low-grade inflammatory status while the adaptive immunity is characterised by an exhaustion of clone-specific antibodies (Ginaldi et al., 2007). In addition, older people are also more at risk of cancers and autoimmune diseases due to increased susceptibility to infection. Older people not only have a reduction in the level of protection against invading pathogens, but they also have slower and less dramatic hypersensitivity reactions (Linton, 2007).

Changes in the thymus

Atrophy of the thymus occurs naturally and progressively with ageing (Ginaldi et al., 2007). With age, productivity of the thymus decreases and it produces fewer new T cells. The thymus decreases in size and contains fewer thymocytes and epithelial cells. Along with the structural decline of the thymus, thymic productivity declines steadily (Hakim and Gress, 2007). The major impact of this ageing change is on the T cells (Meiner and Lueckenotte, 2006). The atrophying thymus affects the production of naïve or virgin T cells so that a decreased number are produced. Accompanying the decrease in naïve T cells are an increased number of memory cells, increased production of cytokines as well as a collection of activated effector cells that occupy T cell space but are unable to work fully as T cells.

T cell function

Cell-mediated immunity decreases with age; lymphocyte function diminishes and is linked to a decline in T cell function. The T cells themselves are also less able to respond and reproduce after exposure to an antigen (Meiner and Lueckenotte, 2006). Fewer T cells are available to respond to the presence of new antigens due to the involution of the thymus. As a result of this, most T cells in older adults have previously been exposed to an antigen (Linton, 2007). The mass of memory T cells diminish and the availability of naïve T cells is also severely reduced leading to a diminished range of available T cells to combat infection.

Basal levels of immune function are maintained although the ability of the immune system to cope with major immunological stressors including chronic or acute infections diminishes (Ginaldi and Sternberg, 2003). However, immune competence may well be severely limited by the decline in naïve T cell numbers (Hakim and Gress, 2007). Older adults have a greater percentage of memory T cells than naïve T cells, both of which have a diminished functional capacity. The immune system in older people therefore responds more slowly to the presence of new and previously encountered infectious agents (Graham et al., 2006).

B cell function

Humoral immunity in older people is affected by B cells producing less immunoglobulin (antibodies) although they do maintain their numbers. However, there is a related decline in hypersensitivity or allergic reactions (Meiner and Lueckenotte, 2006). There is also a loss in the diversity and affinity of immunoglobulin resulting from disruption to lymphocyte production in the lymph nodes (Aw et al., 2007). There is a corresponding decline in the production of antibodies which are crucial to both innate and adaptive immunity (Castle, 2000 in Graham et al., 2006). There are two particular problems resulting from the changes in humoral (specific) immunity in older people. First, responses to antibodies are reduced, the response to vaccines is of a lower titre, the period of protective immunity is shorter and the antibody affinity is lower. Second, there is an increase in the production of autoantibodies, which may lead to the development of autoimmune disorders. The decline in B cell populations contributes to a gradual shift towards B cell populations and responses dominated by antigen experienced memory B cells (Hakim and Gress, 2007).

A primary immune response is where a person is exposed to a particular antigen for the first time. They often succumb to illness while they identify the specific antigen and mount an appropriate immune response. This immunity is not thought to be affected with age (Meiner and Lueckenotte, 2006).

A secondary immune response is where the person is exposed to a previously encountered antigen. Here, they mount a rapid and violent response to the antigen due to the presence and action of memory cells. The overall immune response is generally rapid and violent enough to remove the offending antigen before the person succumbs to illness. This immune response is not as effective in older adults due to the reasons outlined earlier.

Natural killer cells

There does not seem to be a decrease in NK cell activity (Meiner and Lueckenotte, 2006). However, the total number of NK cells increase with advancing age as does the number of NK cells expressing NK receptors (Linton, 2007). However, the function of the NK cells seems to be depressed in older people (Aw et al., 2007). The production of cytokines by activated NK cells is also impaired. In relation to humoral immunity, there is an increase in autoantibodies even though vaccine response diminishes (Linton, 2007). Circulating NK cells increase in the peripheral blood of healthy people who are over 70 years of age when compared to young or middle-aged people. This increase in NK cells in the peripheral blood is linked to a decrease in the number of T cells. The reduced number of T cells decreases cytolysis (destruction of cells) which appears to be compensated for by an increase in the number of NK cells (Ginaldi et al., 2007).

Inflammatory process

There is no doubt that as we age we are increasingly at risk of developing a number of inflammatory disorders including diabetes, sarcopenia and atherosclerosis. The increasing risk of inflammatory disorders in old age may be linked to the fact that people are living much longer than their ancestors and the immune system has to function and protect the individual for a far greater length of time than before (Ginaldi et al., 2007). Therefore, older people are exposed to many years of antigenic stressors. This chronic antigenic stress and subsequent inflammatory burden have a major impact on survival and frailty. The lengthy period of activity of the immune system leads to inflammation which over time becomes chronic and goes on to damage several organs in the body. The process of chronic inflammation that is peculiarly linked to the ageing individual is called inflammaging. The process of inflammaging seems to be under genetic control and has a deleterious effect on longevity. The ageing immune system becomes less able to respond to the effects of new antigens on the one hand, but on the other hand becomes more prone to chronic inflammatory reactions. This pro-inflammatory condition is referred to as chronic antigenic overload (Ginaldi et al., 2007).

As ageing occurs, the production of pro-inflammatory cytokines by macrophages and fibroblasts increases. As compared to younger adults, middle-aged and older adults typically have higher levels of cytokines with pro-inflammatory functions circulating in the blood (Graham et al., 2006). The body is therefore continually challenged by antigens resulting in the production and release of inflammatory mediators which then trigger associated inflammatory diseases (Aw et al., 2007). Inflammatory processes are part of the non-specific immune response. This is evident when acute infection or tissue damage is present and inflammatory processes are triggered in order to isolate the affected area and initiate body responses to begin removal of the offending antigen. The inflammatory response includes increasing the flow of blood to and from the area of inflammation and movement of cells and fluids from blood vessels to the site of inflammation, both of which contribute to redness, heat, swelling and discomfort. Fever can also be associated with inflammation due to the release of pyrogens from white blood cells or from bacterial toxins. Pyrogens are fever-inducing substances.

Pro-inflammatory cytokine proteins enhance communication between the cells that have a central role in the inflammatory process. In older adults, wound healing may be impaired due to reduced ability of macrophages to produce pro-inflammatory cytokines in the local environment.

Chronic inflammation has been described as a dangerous disruption of homeostasis and increases the likelihood of developing long-term conditions such as atherosclerosis, cardiovascular disease, cancer, osteoporosis and rheumatoid arthritis (Graham et al., 2006).

The innate immune system is supported by a number of different factors which are outlined as follows. These supporting factors become less effective with advancing age.

Nutrition

Older people have an increased risk of developing nosocomial infections as a result of under-nutrition, unintentional weight loss and low serum albumin levels (Meiner and Lueckenotte, 2006). Older people who have nutritional deficiencies have considerable reductions in delayed cutaneous hypersensitivity also known as type IV hypersensitivity reactions. A significant deficiency of protein and energy nutrients leads to major alterations in immune function (Carter and Pottinger, 2001). These alterations include impairment of maturing T cells. Serum immunoglobulin G and immunoglobulin M (antibodies) levels are also diminished. There is a decline in the number of phagocytic cells and they no longer function effectively. This allows microorganisms to develop and reproduce more readily. Complement activity is also reduced (Linton, 2007). Complement refers to a group of plasma proteins which, when activated, leads to an action known as 'membrane attack complex'. This action results in the destruction of the invading microorganism.

Complement activity supports the body's defence systems. Overall, these changes lead to an increased risk of infection.

If iron and trace element deficiency are present, there is compromise of lymphocyte and granulocyte functions. Low iron levels decrease the number of circulating T cells and also contribute to a decline in the function of neutrophils, macrophages, B cells and T cells. The functional decline of these defence cells can lead to a delay in the body's response to antigens.

The trace elements zinc, selenium and copper are all necessary for a healthy immune system (Meiner and Lueckenotte, 2006). If zinc deficiency becomes chronic, it may result in impaired cell-mediated immunity, wound healing and protein synthesis (Gorczynski and Terzioglu, 2008). The trace elements selenium and copper also improve humoral immunity. The presence of selenium seems to be implicated in protecting the body against malignancy.

Vitamin deficiencies also affect immune function. Vitamins A, C, D, E and B6 are important for cell-mediated immunity while vitamin C supplements may improve the ability of lymphocytes to respond when required. If dietary supplements of A, C and E are taken, they can improve cell-mediated immunity in older people (Meiner and Lueckenotte, 2006). If there is a deficiency in vitamin E, there appears to be a reduction in the function of NK cells which are essential for immunity against both tumours and viruses (Gorczynski and Terzioglu, 2008).

Unsaturated fats may impair immune function and increase the possibility of the development of autoimmune disease. Polyunsaturated fats have been linked to a decline in T cell function (Meiner and Lueckenotte, 2006).

Activity

Outline an eating plan for older adults that will promote a healthy immune system.

Changes to the skin and mucous membranes

Changes to the skin occur as a result of the ageing process. These skin changes can also affect the immune system. The changes in the skin include a reduction in the amount of circulating thymus-derived lymphocytes, cytokines and epidermal Langerhans cells (Linton, 2007). The Langerhans cells are responsible for immuno-surveillance and can detect and respond to the presence of microbial antigens.

A decrease in immune function affects the skin and mucous membrane barriers in the following manner. There is a decrease in skin turgor, making the skin drier and less acidic. The decrease in skin acidity may allow for easier growth and reproduction of certain bacteria. These changes may also result in the skin breaking down more easily.

There is a reduction in the cough reflex, and the sweeping action of the cilia in the respiratory tract diminishes. These make it more likely for infectious microorganisms to invade and colonise the lungs leading to a number of respiratory infections including pneumonia.

Changes in the urinary system include incomplete bladder emptying, detrusor muscle weakness and prostatic hypertrophy, all of which increase the risk of UTIs. Oestrogen levels diminish, making older women increasingly at risk of UTI and vaginitis. Changes in the digestive system include a reduction in gastric motility. There is also a decrease in acid production which increases the risk of gastro-enteritis or diarrhoea in older people (Gorczynski and Terzioglu, 2008).

HIV/AIDS

In the following section, we will examine HIV/AIDS and consider the implications that this disorder of the immune system has for older adults. Assessment of the immune system will be considered followed by a discussion on HIV/AIDS as an example of a disease that causes an immune deficit. Nursing assessment of the immune system is aimed at identifying the risk to the person of developing infection. As the first line of defence includes the muco-cutaneous barriers, they need to be assessed. Therefore, the assessment is wide ranging and includes a number of body systems. The discussion will also include why older people with HIV and AIDS may not receive the care that they may need.

It is important to acknowledge that the immune system of an older person becomes less efficient as a result of the ageing process; therefore, the classic symptoms of infection may not always be present. There may be a decline in the inflammatory responses which can result in false negatives for skin tests that are used in the diagnosis of a disease. There may be a lack of redness, swelling or inflammation, all of which are normally signs of the presence of infection. Further depression of inflammatory responses may occur if older patients are taking immunosuppressant drugs for another disorder, for example cancer, or they have other diseases that further depress the immune system. The absence of fever can be another change relating to the ageing immune system so that the temperature either does not rise in the presence of infection or it rises minimally. Symptoms of pain may also be absent or reduced.

Due to the lack of typical signs and symptoms of infection, an older person may be critically ill before an infection is identified and acted upon. If an older person has signs of low-grade pyrexia, then efforts should be made to find its source, as it may be a precursor to severe illness. Other signs and symptoms that are indicative of infection in older adults include malaise or fatigue, and if these are combined with other symptoms of illness, the patient should be examined for the presence of infection (Thames and Meiner, 2006). However, white blood cell count will still increase in the presence of infection (Soule et al., 1995) unless the patient is on immunosuppressants.

Assessment of the immune system

A full health history should be taken and which may include the following questions
(Adapted from Linton, 2007; Meiner and Lueckenotte, 2006)

- Has the patient had any recent, recurrent or chronic infections? (Linton, 2007).
- If so, how severe was the infection, when did it occur and where was the infection? Due to the reduced immune response associated with ageing older adults on second exposure to the same antigen, the older adult may not be able to mount the typical rapid

and extremely violent immune response and as a result may succumb to infection again (Thames and Meiner, 2006). A younger person's response following exposure to the same antigen is generally rapid and violent enough to remove the offending microorganism before symptoms of infection.

- Has the patient had cancer or is being treated for cancer, liver or kidney disorders?
- Has the patient been diagnosed with HIV infection or any autoimmune disorders?
- Has the patient been in a situation where they may have been engaged in risk taking activities with people who are HIV positive?
- Has the patient had delayed wound healing?
- Has the patient experienced any problems with prolonged bleeding before?
- Has the patient had any blood transfusions? If so, when and where?
- Does the patient have an intravenous cannula *in situ*?
- Does the patient have a urinary catheter *in situ*?
- Is the patient complaining of fatigue or general malaise?
- Does the patient complain of fevers, chills or night sweats?
- Are there any skin lesions, evidence of itch, bleeding or bruising?
- Does the patient have a headache?
- Does the patient have a sore throat?
- Are there any respiratory symptoms?
- Is the patient's nutritional intake satisfactory? Is there any evidence of under-nutrition or weight changes?
- Does the patient have enlarged lymph nodes?
- Has there been any change in bowel habits?
- Are there any urinary symptoms including dysuria or haematuria?
- What medications does the patient take including prescription and over-the-counter medications?
- Is the patient an intravenous drug user? Is there a history of sharing needles?
- Does the patient drink more than moderate levels of alcohol?
- Information about sexual activity relating to partners, number of partners and the use of condoms if necessary.
- How much exercise does the patient take?
- Have they had any stressors lately, for example, bereavement or moving house?

Physical examination would include temperature, pulse, blood pressure, respiratory rate, oxygen saturation, urinalysis, stool sample, sputum sample if necessary. The patient's skin and mucous membranes should be assessed and the size of lymph nodes should be checked.

General advice for people who are caring for older adults at risk of infection due to changes in the immune system include:

- Implementation of strict infection control procedures.
- Ensure that older people are advised about the importance of immunisations.
- If the patient is in hospital, relatives who have respiratory infections should be advised not to visit until they are recovered.
- Nurses need to consider carefully whether the use of a urinary catheter is necessary for each older patient.

- Older people should be encouraged to drink at least 1500–2000 ml of fluids every day.
- Hygiene standards should be rigorously maintained.

(Adapted from Thames and Meiner, 2006)

Nutrition and exercise are very important for the maintenance of a healthy immune system. A nutritious diet with adequate amounts of carbohydrate, proteins and fats, sufficient vitamins and trace minerals including iron, zinc, selenium and copper will help improve immune responses (Thames and Meiner, 2006). Antioxidants help to break down free radicals which are thought to be important in the prevention of the development of cancer. Kohut et al. (2004) suggests that moderate exercise over time boosts the immune response.

HIV/AIDS

Human immunodeficiency virus is a member of the retrovirus family that can lead to the development of AIDS. Upon entry to a host cell, the retroviral RNA is converted to double-stranded DNA by the action of the enzyme reverse transcriptase. The viral DNA is now inserted into the host cell's DNA by the action of another enzyme, integrase, and in this way the viral DNA is incorporated into the substance of the host cell's DNA. This can permit the virus to 'hijack' the cell in order to produce multiple new viral particles. The virus can enter a dormant phase or can become active immediately and begin replicating new particles. Following replication of virus, the new virus particles are released from the host cell and infect surrounding cells.

Human immunodeficiency virus infects cells of the immune system and central nervous system (CNS). The cells involved in the immune system are the helper T cells. Helper T cells activate and direct the actions of other immune cells and are involved in the coordination of the overall immune response. Helper T cells are targeted by HIV because they have a particular protein found on their surface membrane called CD4. This is the protein that HIV attaches to before entering the cell. Other cells in the body with CD4 on their surface membranes are also targeted by HIV.

When the number of helper T cells is reduced through the action of HIV, the immune system is less able to protect the body and the person becomes susceptible to opportunistic infections. It may take several years before the person's immune system is substantially weakened through the loss of number of T cells.

Stages of HIV infection

There are four distinct stages of infection in HIV – acute, asymptomatic, late stage (pre-AIDS), late stage (AIDS).

Modes of transmission related to older adults

Contact with infected blood/blood products:

- Transfusions with infected blood
- Sharing of needles or syringes between infected individuals

- Percutaneous needlestick injury
- Body piercing or tattooing using unsanitary techniques.

Sexual contact:

- Unprotected vaginal or anal intercourse is the most common means of transmission.

There are many reasons why a number of older people are at risk of developing HIV and AIDS. The increasing availability of drugs similar to sildenafil (Viagra) have revolutionised older men's lives if they have been experiencing penile dysfunction. The divorce rates among older people have risen so that they are more likely to have more than one partner and people reaching old age now are more sexually liberated than previous cohorts (Dougan et al., 2004). The cohorts that are going in to old age may include people who have a history of intravenous drug use. Other risk factors include contact with commercial sex workers. Furthermore, older women are less likely to use contraceptives. Age-related changes in the vagina, such as thinning of vaginal walls, vaginal pH becoming more alkaline and lack of lubrication, also increase the susceptibility to trauma and disease. Global travel is another factor and older travellers may engage in risky behaviours when removed from their normal environment (Linton, 2007). People diagnosed with HIV or AIDS are now living longer due to successful treatment with highly active antiretroviral therapy (HAART). The mean age of diagnosis of HIV is also rising.

Dougan et al. (2004) carried out a prevalence study to identify how many older people develop AIDS and the most likely causative routes of infection. In line with many studies, the definition of old age starts at a younger age than is usually used. They defined an older individual as 45 or over. Fourteen per cent of newly diagnosed people with AIDS were aged 45 or older. Of those people, 69% ranged from 45 to 54; 25% from 55 to 64; 6.4% between 65 and above. Sex between men and women accounted for 47% of infections diagnosed in older individuals, while 45% of new diagnoses in older individuals were acquired through homosexual activities. A small number of older individuals developed HIV through injecting drugs and through blood transfusions. Twenty-six per cent of older adults were diagnosed late after the onset of infection, while between the periods of 1997 and 2001 58% had died within 3 months of diagnosis.

Issues relating to older people and HIV/AIDS

Older people are more likely to be misdiagnosed than younger people, as there may be difficulties in differentiating between symptoms that occur in relation to diseases that are common in older age (Dougan et al., 2004).

Ageist perceptions persist where older people are not viewed as sexually active, nor as being as likely to experiment in their sexual activities. These attitudes have excluded older people from surveys regarding sexual attitudes and lifestyles. Many safe sex messages are aimed at younger adults, therefore older adults do not necessarily relate to these messages nor do they assimilate the information. Therefore, older people are less likely to see themselves at risk for HIV infection. Older people may not know how HIV is transmitted, they may be unaware of the risk of HIV and there is a lack of information given to older people from health professionals about how HIV is transmitted (Savasta, 2004). Older people who are aware of the risk factors for the development of HIV may be reluctant to identify that they have put themselves at risk of HIV (Redfern and Ross, 2006). Dougan et al. (2004) in their study identified that older people exhibited higher levels of delaying behaviours compared to younger adults when attending the genito-urinary department. Older people may be reluctant to initiate discussions about their sexual activity while older women are less likely to use condoms with new partners as they are not at risk of pregnancy.

Older adults are more likely to be diagnosed with HIV at a later stage than younger adults, usually after onset of symptoms. Older people experience a speedy immunological decline, and they progress more quickly from HIV status to AIDS. Once the diagnosis of AIDS has been made, older people have a shorter survival time (Valcour et al., 2004). Therefore, for many older adults, there is only a short time interval between the diagnosis of HIV infection to the development of AIDS and death. This is due to the ageing immune system not being able to remove the HIV which has infected macrophages, lymphoid tissue or the brain. Since the immune system loses its ability to regenerate and not all replacement cells are fully functional, the disease progresses more speedily (Adler et al., 1997).

Older people often have co-morbidities that can make the disease process and its management more complex, resulting in increased morbidity and premature mortality (Dolder et al., 2004). Administration of HAART has increased the likelihood of young people who have been diagnosed with HIV surviving into middle age and older age (Redfern and Ross, 2006).

Symptoms of HIV are typical no matter the age, but older people are much more likely to report fewer symptoms. There are two main reasons for this: first, older people may have other disorders which give rise to similar symptoms. Second, symptoms may be related to medication reactions. The symptoms of fatigue, anorexia, weight loss, chronic pain, rash, itching can be interpreted in these ways (Forte et al., 2006). Decreased survival times are common in older people, but this may be linked to the diagnosis being made when the disease is advanced or to the changes in the immune system which have previously been described as immuno-senescence (Linton, 2007). If the disease has advanced prior to diagnosis, HAART is much less effective (Linton, 2007).

Neurological symptoms are varied and may include cognitive, behavioural and psychomotor disturbances. However, other common causes of neurological changes need to be investigated to rule them out. An example of this would be Parkinson's disease (PD) where motor symptoms are similar. HIV-associated dementia seems to be common among HIV-positive older people. HIV/AIDS-related dementia will imitate Alzheimer's disease but there are differences in onset which is sudden for HIV-related dementia, it comes and goes and it may be associated with parkinsonian-type symptoms (Forte et al., 2006).

Opportunistic infections commonly found in HIV are more likely to develop due to less efficient immune systems relating to the ageing process. Commonly found infections include *Pneumocystis carinii* pneumonia (PCP) tuberculosis, oral and genital candidiasis and herpes zoster. The presence of any of these infections should alert health professionals to the possibility of a diagnosis of HIV in older people. Similarly, if an older person is diagnosed with non-Hodgkin's lymphoma or Kaposi's sarcoma, the health professional should rule out the possibility of a diagnosis of AIDS.

When working with older people universal precautions should always be taken. However, this is not always the case when attending to the older adult as many health professionals do not consider that older people may be HIV positive (Forte et al., 2006).

Measures to manage HIV symptoms and the adverse effects of treatments are no different for older people than for younger people. These measures include:

- Infection control procedures
- Management of medications
- Education about the common signs and symptoms of infection
- The implications of having HIV on roles and relationships and lifestyle changes to manage the disease
- An understanding of the pathophysiology of the disease
- Support for the family and for the informal carers
- The offer of support groups and counselling
- The provision of an atmosphere of acceptance
- Factual information about progress and prognosis of the disease
- Encourage decision making about their own care and management.

(Adapted from Linton, 2007)

It should be noted that HIV/AIDS services ought to be tailored to meet the needs of older people (Linsk et al., 2003).

Activity

Imagine you have been asked to give a sexual health talk to a group of older adults. List the topics that you may wish to include.

Summary

In this chapter, we have examined the role that the immune system has to play in protecting us from harm. A health immune system protects us from pathogenic microorganisms, thus limiting the damage caused by local and systemic infections. The immune system also participates in the necessary removal of dead or damaged cells and tissues within the body.

Acute inflammation is a normal protective response in a healthy person; however, inflammation can become problematic if it becomes a chronic state of affairs. Older adults may suffer from chronic inflammatory problems such as atherosclerosis and arthritis.

The importance of a balanced and healthy diet in maintaining a healthy immune system cannot be over emphasised. Chapter 6 contains additional information on what such a diet for an older person should consist of. Similarly, healthy, intact skin and mucous membranes are necessary as a first-line defence in preventing the entry of potentially harmful microorganisms into the body.

We suspect that many of you will be surprised at the choice of HIV/AIDS as the health issue which we chose to focus on in this chapter. Hopefully, now that you have worked your way through it, you can now appreciate why this is considered to be a growing issue in older adult care. Health-care professionals need a sound knowledge base in respect of HIV/AIDS in order to respond to client/patient queries and to ensure that the topic of HIV/AIDS is not seen as a problem of only younger client groups.

References and further reading

Adler, W.H., Baskar, P.V., Chrest, F.J., Dorsey-Cooper, B., Winchurch, R.A. and Nagel, J.E. 1997. HIV infection and aging: mechanisms to explain the accelerated rate of progression in the older patient. Mechanical Aging and Development 96, 137–155.

Aw, D., Silva, B. and Palmer, D. 2007. Immunosenescence: emerging challenges for an ageing population. Immunology 120, 435–446.

Carter, C. and Pottinger, J. 2001. Risk for infection. In Maas, M., Buckwalter, K., Hardy, M., Tripp-Reimer, T., Titler, M. and Specht, J. (Eds). Nursing Care of Older Adults. Diagnosis, Outcomes and Interventions. Mosby, St. Louis, MO.

Dolder, C., Patterson, T. and Jeste, D. 2004. HIV, psychosis and ageing: past, present and future. AIDS 81(Suppl. 1), S35–S42.

Dougan, S., Payne, L.J.C., Brown, A.E., Evans, B.G. and Gill, O.N. 2004. Past it? HIV in older people in England, Wales and Northern Ireland. Epidemiology Infections 132, 1151–1160.

Forte, D., Cotter, A. and Wells, D. 2006. Sexuality and relationships in later life. In Redfern, S. and Ross, F. (Eds). Nursing Older People. 4th ed. Churchill Livingstone, Edinburgh.

Ginaldi, L. and Sternberg, H. 2003. The immune system. In Timiras, P. (Ed). Physiological Basis of Aging and Geriatrics. 3rd ed. CRC Press, Boca Raton, FL.

Ginaldi, L., Mengoli, L. and De Martinis, M. 2007. Review on immunosenescence. Review in Clinical Gerontology 17, 161–169.

Gorczynski, R. and Terzioglu, E. 2008. Aging in the immune system. International Urology and Nephrology 40, 1117–1125.

Graham, J., Christian, L. and Kiecolt-Glaser, J. 2006. Stress, age, and immune function: toward a lifespan approach. Journal of Behavioural Medicine 29(4), 389–400.

Hakim, F. and Gress, R. 2007. Immunosenescence. Tissue Antigens 70, 179–189.

Kohut, M., Arnston, B., Lee, B., et al. 2004. Moderate exercise improved antibody response to influenza immunization in older adults. Vaccine 22, 17–18.

Linsk, N.L., Fowler, J.P. and Klein, S.J. 2003. HIV/AIDS prevention and care services and services for the aging: bridging the gap between service systems to assist older people. Journal of Acquired Immune Deficiency Syndromes 33, 243–250.

Linton, A. 2007. Immune system. In Linton, A. and Lach, H. (Eds). Matteson and McConnell's Gerontological Nursing Concepts and Practice. 3rd ed. Saunders Elsevier, Philadelphia, PA.

Meiner, S.E. and Lueckenotte, A.G. 2006. Gerontologic Nursing. 3rd ed. Mosby Elsevier, St. Louis, MO.

Redfern, S. and Ross, F. 2006. Nursing Older People. 4th ed. Churchill Livingstone, Edinburgh.

Savasta, A. 2004. HIV: associated transmission risks in older adults – an integrative review of the literature. Journal of the Association of Nurses in AIDS Care 15(1), 50–59.

Soule, B., Larson, E. and Preston, G. 1995. Infections and Nursing Practice. Mosby, St. Louis, MO.

Thames, D. and Meiner, S. 2006. Infection. In Meiner, S. and Lueckenotte, A. (Eds). Gerontological Nursing. 3rd ed. Mosby Elsevier, St. Louis, MO.

Tortora, G. 2005. Principals of Human Anatomy. 10th ed. Wiley, Hoboken, NJ.

Valcour, V., Shikuma, C., Watters, M., et al. 2004. Age, lipoprotein E4, and the risk of HIV dementia: the Hawaii aging with HIV cohort. Journal of Neuroimmunology 157, 197–202.

Useful websites

Centre for Aids Prevention Studies. http://www.caps.ucsf.edu/pubs/FS/over50.php.

The Body. The complete HIV/AIDS resource. http://www.thebody.com/index/whatis/older.html.

Chapter 4

Communicating

Aims

After reading this chapter you will be able to discuss the structure and function of the nervous system and special senses and relate this to the activity of communicating.

Learning Outcomes

After completion of this chapter you will be able to:

- Describe the normal structure and function of the nervous system and the special senses
- Conduct a comprehensive patient assessment of the above systems using appropriate tools
- Detail the changes in the above systems that are associated with ageing
- Discuss the presentation and management of some common health problems related to the above systems that occur in older adults.

Introduction

This chapter will begin with an overview of the normal anatomy and physiology of the nervous system and special senses pertinent to communication. We will then consider ageing changes in relation to the nervous system and the structures associated with the special senses. We then go on to discuss the effects these changes have on the older person's ability to communicate effectively.

Neurological assessment tools will be described and discussed in relation to their use with older people. This will include assessment of hearing and vision.

The Physiological Effects of Ageing: Implications for Nursing Practice, First Edition
© Alistair Farley, Ella McLafferty and Charles Hendry
Published 2011 by Blackwell Publishing Ltd

Common problems encountered when communicating with older people will be identified. For example, this will include problems associated with the special senses such as conductive deafness and presbyopia. Parkinson's disease (PD) will be considered as it can affect all types of communication, namely verbal and written communications, facial expressions and body language. We will also examine, in detail, the impact that episodes of delirium may have on an older person's capacity to communicate.

This chapter also discusses the support older patients require in relation to communicating both in the community and in hospital settings. This chapter will conclude by discussing the nursing interventions that a health-care professional may utilise in order to assist older adults to continue to communicate effectively.

Normal structure and function

The nervous system

The human body systems which detect and respond to changes in the internal and external environment are:

- The nervous system
- The endocrine system.

We will not consider the endocrine system further in this chapter as the focus on this chapter is those systems and organs that are specifically concerned with the activity of communication.

General structure

The central nervous system (CNS) consists of the brain and spinal cord, and the peripheral nervous system (PNS) is comprised of those nerves which lie outside the CNS (Figure 4.1). These nerves are either afferent nerves which detect and transmit information towards the CNS or efferent nerves which are carrying information away from the CNS.

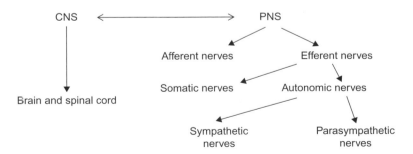

Figure 4.1   Component parts of nervous system.

Efferent nerves are further divided into somatic nerves (those under voluntary control) and autonomic nerves (not under voluntary control). The autonomic nerves are also divided into two types – sympathetic nerves (which generally prepare the body for action) and parasympathetic nerves (normally associated with rest and digestive functions).

Neurones

The functional cells of the nervous system are called neurones. There are about 12 billion of these functional cells in the brain, spinal cord and nerves. They are capable of transmitting impulses to and from all parts of the body.

Some neurones are very short, having to transmit impulses extremely short distances within the brain, while some are very long such as those which transmit impulses from the spinal cord to the feet. In addition, various types of supporting cells are found in the CNS and the PNS where they nourish, protect and insulate neurones (Seeley et al., 2003). These cells, called neuroglia, do not transmit nervous impulses. Schwann cells are an example of neuroglia and are found wrapped around many of the axons in the PNS. These cells insulate and protect the axons in the PNS. They also speed up the rate at which nerve impulses are transmitted.

The brain

The brain lies within the cranial cavity of the skull, where it is surrounded by fluid, membranes and bones for protection. It consists of:

- Cerebrum
- Cerebellum
- Diencephalon
- Brainstem.

Cerebrum

The cerebrum is the structure that most people think of when they think of the brain. It is divided into two hemispheres. The motor nerves in each hemisphere control the opposite side of the body. The two hemispheres are internally connected by white matter containing axons connecting the two hemispheres, known as the corpus callosum. These connections allow for communication between the two hemispheres and contribute to, for example, the coordination of movement and the ability to think about complex information.

The surface (or cortex) of the cerebrum is convoluted by folds called gyri and grooves called sulci. The convolutions greatly increase the surface area of the brain in order to accommodate the neuronal cell bodies (which form the grey matter of the brain) which process and integrate information and initiate responses. Without this greatly increased surface area, we could only fit a brain of about one-third the size into the cranial cavity with a corresponding loss of processing power (Saladin, 2001).

Revision Point

Identify where in the brain you can find the following functional areas:

- Visual cortex
- Motor cortex
- Speech cortex
- Sensory cortex
- Auditory centres
- Centre for behaviour and motivation.

The basal nuclei (ganglia) are paired masses of grey matter which lie deep within the cerebral hemispheres. They help to plan, and control muscular movements and posture (Seeley et al., 2005). Damage to the basal nuclei can cause movement disorders such as PD. As we will see later, this disease can impact on a person's ability to communicate.

Cerebellum

The cerebellum is situated posterior to the medulla oblongata and the pons varolii and inferior to the cerebrum. It is similar in structure to the cerebrum, that is, convoluted on the surface and divided into two hemispheres. The cerebellum is involved in maintaining balance, muscle tone and coordinated movement. It does this together with the cerebrum and basal ganglia.

Diencephalon

The diencephalon lies between the cerebrum and brainstem. It consists of several structures including the thalamus and hypothalamus. The thalamus acts as a relay station for most sensory input before the impulse reaches the sensory cortex. The hypothalamus has several important functions outlined as follows:

- Regulation of homeostasis (constancy within the body)
- Autonomic nervous system (ANS) and endocrine system regulation
- Temperature regulation (thermostat)
- Regulates thirst, hunger and satiety (sense of fullness)
- Regulates emotional responses such as anger, fear, pain and pleasure
- Regulates behavioural patterns in relation to sexual arousal
- Regulates sleeping and wakefulness.

Limbic system

The limbic system is found within the cerebrum and diencephalon and it is, together with the hypothalamus, involved in regulating emotional behaviours such as pain, pleasure and anger. Emotions such as these are often largely communicated using non-verbal means such as facial expression and gestures.

Table 4.1   Vital centres located in the medulla oblongata.

Centre	Regulates
Cardiac centre	Heart rate and stroke volume
Respiratory centre (in addition to that located in the pons)	Breathing patterns
Vasomotor centre	Blood pressure
Reflex centres	Coughing, sneezing and vomiting

Brainstem

The brainstem consists of the midbrain, the pons varolii and the medulla oblongata.

The midbrain is composed mainly of nerve tracts passing to and from the brain and spinal cord. It also contains cells involved in eye movements, pupil diameter, the startle reflex and the reflex of turning the head to loud noise or bright light.

The pons contains nervous connections between the cerebrum and cerebellum. It also contains nuclei whose function is to regulate breathing.

The medulla oblongata is the most inferior part of the brainstem and continues inferiorly with the spinal cord (Seeley et al., 2003). It contains ascending and descending nerve fibres as well as a number of cranial nerve nuclei (see section on Cranial Nerves), other nuclei and part of the reticular system. It is an area in which nerves descending from the brain cross over to the opposite side, thus allowing one side of the brain to influence the other side of the body. This also explains how damage to one side of the brain can produce clinical features of disorder on the opposite of the body, as in stroke. The medulla also contains several important 'vital centres' which ensure that key physiological functions are maintained. These are indicated in Table 4.1.

The reticular activating system (RAS) is found in the brainstem. This area of the CNS helps to maintain consciousness and is involved in the regulation of the 'sleep–wake cycle'. Activation of the RAS generally leads to wakefulness, whereas inactivation of the RAS produces sleep.

The spinal cord

The spinal cord lies in the vertebral canal and runs from the brainstem to the level of the second lumbar vertebra. Thirty-one pairs of spinal nerves enter and leave the spinal cord down its length. It is composed of cervical, thoracic, lumbar and sacral segments, taking their name from the part of the vertebral column at which their nerves enter and exit. The spinal cord is shorter than the vertebral column because the former does not grow as fast during development. Sensory nerves carrying information from the body to the brain enter the posterior part of the spinal cord. Motor nerves carrying information to the body from the brain leave the anterior part of the spinal cord.

Internally, the spinal cord is composed of grey matter (cell bodies) found in columns and arranged in an H shape with white matter (nerve pathways) found in tracts surrounding this. A central canal runs down the middle of the cord. This contains a small amount of cerebrospinal fluid. The spinal cord exits the skull at the opening in the base known as the foramen magnum.

The posterior (dorsal) horns of the H shape manage sensory information entering the CNS from the body. The cell body of the sensory neurones lie outside the spinal cord in the posterior root ganglion. The anterior (ventral) horns of the H shape manage motor information leaving the CNS to have an effect on the body.

The axon of a sensory neurone enters the posterior horn of the spinal cord and synapses (interconnects) with another sensory neurone, the axon of which passes up sensory pathways in the spinal cord to the brain. Following interpretation of this information, the axon of a motor neurone passes down the motor pathway in the spinal cord. At the appropriate level in the spinal cord, the first motor neurone will synapse with a second motor neurone in the anterior horn of the spinal cord, and the axon of this neurone then forms the motor nerve. The neurone from the brain down the motor pathway of the spinal cord (first motor neurone) is known as the upper motor neurone, and the neurone from the spinal cord to the muscle (second motor neurone) is the lower motor neurone.

Reflex arc

Most of the impulses arriving at the spinal cord from the peripheral nerves are transmitted to the brain for interpretation and action. However, when the sensory neurones entering the spinal cord interpret a signal as dangerous (e.g. touching a hot surface, standing on a nail), a message is transmitted across the spinal cord to a motor neurone from where the message can be directed straight to a muscle bringing about the action of removing the body from danger. This is called a reflex action and happens without conscious control. At the same time as the reflex is happening, messages are being transmitted up the spinal cord to the brain so that you become aware of the action after it has happened.

Protection of the nervous system

The brain and spinal cord are protected by the bones of the skull and vertebral column, soft tissue membranes known as the meninges and cerebrospinal fluid. The meninges are a triple layer of tissue surrounding the brain and spinal cord. The outermost layer is the dura mater, the middle layer is known as the arachnoid mater and the inner layer is the pia mater. Between the arachnoid and pia mater is a space known as the sub-arachnoid space which contains cerebrospinal fluid. This fluid acts as a shock absorber, further protecting the brain and spinal cord.

Blood supply

Like every other tissue, nervous tissue must have a supply of oxygen and nutrients in order to produce energy for transmitting impulses. The right and left vertebral arteries originate from a major branch of the aorta. On the underside of the brain, they unite to form the basilar artery.

The right and left internal carotids also originate from the aorta. Within the skull, they unite with the basilar artery to form the circle of Willis. Arteries arising from this circle supply the brain with oxygenated blood. The main veins which return blood to the heart from the brain are the internal jugular veins.

Cranial and spinal nerves

Cranial nerves pass to and from the brain and brainstem through holes in the skull. All but one (the vagus or 10th cranial nerve) are concerned with sensation and/or function of the head and neck.

 Revision Point

Identify the 12 cranial nerves and their function.

The autonomic nervous system

The CNS is responsible for allowing voluntary control, that is, the things we choose to do or not, for example, sitting, standing, walking, chewing. The ANS is responsible for involuntary control, that is, the things that go on in the body which are not normally under voluntary control but help to maintain homeostasis, such as digestion, control of blood pressure, regulation of body temperature, regulation of amount of light entering the eye and so on.

The ANS has two divisions, namely:

1. Sympathetic division which has a major effect under conditions of stress and activity and prepares the body for action in order to maintain homeostasis. This is known as the 'fight or flight' response.
2. Parasympathetic division which is responsible for the day-to-day maintenance of homeostasis largely through rest and digestive functions.

In many organs, the two divisions work in cooperation having the opposite effects in order to maintain homeostasis despite changes in circumstances.

 Revision Point

Determine the effects stimulation by the sympathetic and parasympathetic divisions of the ANS will have on the following:

- Heart rate
- Respiratory rate
- Pupil size
- Digestion.

The CNS and ANS work closely together and many structures of the CNS also contain functional parts of the ANS.

Ageing changes in the nervous system

Brain

When healthy, the ageing brain continues to function normally throughout old age. The brain is able to adapt and compensate for any cellular and neuronal changes brought about by the ageing process and an older person remains able to learn during old age. However, the ageing process does affect the different cells and functions of the brain in different ways (Timiras, 2003). Timiras goes on to state that healthy older people seem to display no significant differences when examined using imaging techniques for the weight, size, volume and metabolism of the brain as compared to younger people.

The meninges which surround the brain thicken with age. The dura mater, which is the outer layer of the meninges, holds fast to the skull in very old adults. The blood vessels in the arachnoid layer reflect the vascular condition of the rest of the body (Christiansen and Grzybowski, 1999). This is also reflected in the cerebral blood flow as it diminishes with age. However, the amount of oxygen which is delivered to the brain remains adequate as a result of more oxygen being released from haemoglobin, as increased amounts of oxygen are extracted from the blood (Redfern and Ross, 2001).

There appears to be some shrinkage of the healthy brain during ageing but it does not seem to have any significant effect on an older person's brain function, including the ability to continue learning (Timiras, 2003). Brain weight declines from $\sim$1400 g in a typical young male adult to about 1200–1300 g in very old adults. Until the age of 50, there appears to be only a small amount of brain weight loss; however, this loss speeds up after the age of 60 (Christiansen and Grzybowski, 1999). Timiras (2003) accounts for the change in the brain weight as a result of the loss of neurones. However, Lueckenotte (2000) suggests that the decrease in brain weight may be due to a reduction in the size of some neurones rather than the loss of neurones.

The loss of brain weight is accompanied by alterations in the appearance and organisation of the brain (Christiansen and Grzybowski, 1999). The gyri flatten and decrease in size while the sulci widen and deepen, resulting in a decrease in the cortical area in the brain. Interestingly, this loss of hemispheric volume occurs at a faster rate in men than in women (Linton and Matteson, 1997). The general shrinkage of brain size results in increased separation from the skull and an increase in the size of the ventricles (Christiansen and Grzybowski, 1999; Linton and Matteson, 1997). Loss of lipid-rich myelin also occurs, resulting in an increase in water and protein content of the brain (Linton and Matteson, 1997).

Neuronal loss

There seems to be a steady loss of neurones in the brain and spinal cord with ageing. At the age of 75, the loss is estimated to be about 10%. However, because there are very large numbers of neurones in the brain, this progressive loss of neurones does not result in a significant loss of mental functioning (Roach, 2001).

Loss of neurones appears to be patchy and affects only some areas of the brain. Neuronal loss also seems to vary from individual to individual. In some areas of the cerebral cortex and in the cerebellum, the number of neurones remains virtually unchanged throughout life, except when people become very old and loss then starts to appear in the cerebellum. Neuronal losses do occur in the locus caeruleus (an area of the brainstem concerned with the physiological response to stress and panic) where catecholaminergic neurones are found, the substantia nigra where dopaminergic neurones are found, the nucleus basalis of Meynert (NBM) and the hippocampus where cholinergic neurones are found. Overall, neuronal loss seems to be fairly small. However, a severe loss of cholinergic neurones or loss of dopaminergic neurones has to occur before the development of Alzheimer's disease or PD becomes apparent, respectively.

There seems to be a steady loss of neurones with ageing. However, once lost, neurones are not replaced with other neurones. They are replaced with cells known as neuroglial cells, which do not directly influence electrical impulse transmission (Linton and Matteson, 1997). This increase in number of neuroglial (glial) cells is a normal compensatory response to ageing changes in the CNS (Timiras, 2003). However, the number of neuronal cells in the brainstem remains fairly constant into old age. This is significant due to the presence of many vital centres found within the brainstem (Redfern and Ross, 2001).

Neuronal networks

Organisation of neuronal networks is preserved in healthy older people. However, with continued advancing age, the number of dendrites and dendritic branches may decrease. The reduction of dendrites and dendritic branches can result in isolation of neurones and a slowing down or failure of communication between neurones. However, as dendrites undergo continuous renewal throughout their lifespan, the reduction in the number of dendrites may not reflect an actual loss but reflect a slowing down of the renewal process (Timiras, 2003). In areas of the CNS where numbers of dendrites and their branches reduce, there is also a decrease in numbers of synapses. Attempts are made to compensate for this loss by increasing the number of synapses provided by surrounding neurones (Timiras, 2003). There is an increase in dendritic growth in some neurones found in the cerebral cortex and hippocampus. This increase may be associated with an attempt to compensate for neuronal loss in specific areas of the brain (Linton and Matteson, 1997).

With advancing age, a number of changes occur in neurones including a reduction in RNA, mitochondria and enzymes contained within the cytoplasm. The size of nuclei also decreases. Axons degenerate, swell and lose myelin – a process known as dying back. Dendrite changes affect synaptic transmissions as do changes in neurotransmitters (Linton and Matteson, 1997).

Neurotransmitters

Neuronal activity slows down with advancing age. This slowing down is related to the lowered production and metabolism of the main neurotransmitters, especially where nerve conduction is across multi-synaptic junctions (Linton and Matteson, 1997). In healthy older people, neurotransmitter levels and activities undergo minor changes only. Timiras (2003) suggests that functional ability of older adults can be altered due to a loss of balance between excitatory and inhibitory neurotransmitters. An example of such imbalance can be seen in PD where levels of the inhibitory neurotransmitter dopamine decline but levels of the excitatory neurotransmitter acetylcholine remains the same. Due to this change in balance between these two neurotransmitters, one of the most notable features of PD – tremor – is experienced. A decline in norepinephrine has also been found and lower levels of dopamine have been measured especially in the basal ganglia of older people (Christiansen and Grzybowski, 1999).

Lipofuscin and neurofibrillary tangles

Many CNS cells in the older adult contain considerable quantities of the yellow/brown pigment known as lipofuscin. This pigment is linked to the accumulation of free radicals within a number of body cells including cells in heart muscle and in the skin. Lipofuscin is thought to be derived from waste products from partially broken down cell membranes and other cell structures. These wastes are thought to cram the cytoplasm resulting in less effective cellular work (Lueckenotte, 2000). Accumulation of this pigment is part of the normal ageing process and found within the normal ageing brain (Christiansen and Grzybowski, 1999).

Neurofibrillary tangles are insoluble twisted fibres found within cells of the brain. They are composed of a protein known as tau which forms part of a structure called a microtubule. These tangles are found within the cells of the brain as part of the normal ageing process (Redfern and Ross, 2001; Timiras, 2003). However, they are also found within neurones of patients diagnosed with Alzheimer's disease.

Movement

In most healthy older adults, there is no noticeable loss of cognition. However, there is a degree of loss in sensory function due to the loss of sensory neurones. This can result in impairment of hearing, vision, smelling, temperature regulation and pain sensation (Roach, 2001). Loss of postural control is influenced by the loss of sensory cues, especially visual, tactile and auditory cues. These losses contribute to the increased risk of falls in many older adults. Slower reflexes associated with ageing are common as is a delayed response to stimuli. These changes are related to a reduction in the number of nerve conduction fibres (Roach, 2001). Overall reaction time is slower but older adults are generally aware of this and seem to compensate by responding more slowly but more precisely (Linton and Matteson, 1997). Given time, older people are capable of performing many tasks as good as younger people.

> **Activity**
>
> Consider the environment in which you work or live. Overall, does it help or hinder the movement of older adults? What changes might make it safer?

Changes in the spinal cord

Changes in nerve cells in the spinal cord are similar to the changes found in the brain. By the age of 90, 30–50% of anterior horn cells are lost and 30% of myelinated axons in the posterior roots and peripheral nerves are lost. Larger nerve fibres are lost in the sympathetic chain, which are thought to account for the increased incidence of postural hypotension in older age. The efferent system that carries information away from the CNS also loses its largest fibres, resulting in slower conduction of nerve impulses.

The overall efficiency of the ANS is reduced with advancing age. Loss of nerve cells, slower conduction of nerve impulses and deterioration in peripheral nerve functions all lead to a decrease in its efficiency. Recovery from stress takes longer than before and is often incomplete. Stressors such as heat, cold and extreme exercise can be particularly harmful and even life-threatening (Linton and Matteson, 1997).

There are also changes in the peripheral nerves associated with ageing. Some axons lose their myelin sheath and Schwann cells may become less efficient or cease to function altogether. It is important to recall that Schwann cells insulate the axon of a nerve cell and also speed up the rate of nerve impulse conduction.

Nerve cells and processes in the spinal cord are also lost as the person ages. Over time these nerve cells are replaced with glial cells in a process called gliosis. Deep tendon reflexes deteriorate with age and many reflexes are lost by the age of 90 (Christiansen and Grzybowski, 1999).

With ageing, many tissues and organs respond less well to sympathetic stimulation. Cardiovascular and blood pressure reflexes are significantly reduced with ageing (Redfern and Ross, 2001), making older adults more prone to problems associated with sudden changes in body positions. An example being postural hypotension, where the vasoconstriction reflexes are not quick enough to maintain systolic blood pressure as a person moves from a sitting or lying position to a standing position. If the vasoconstrictor reflexes are not responsive enough, the person may experience dizziness, light-headedness and blurred vision. This also increases the likelihood of falls.

The vertebral arteries supplying blood to the brain tend to become more tortuous with ageing as a result of changes in the cervical vertebrae and intervertebral discs. Specific movements of the neck can make them kink which can temporarily reduce the supply of blood to the brain. Cerebral arteries and capillaries normally have thinner middle and outer layers compared to other arteries in the body. As with other arteries throughout the body, cerebral arteries are also prone to developing atherosclerotic changes associated with ageing. However, the brain is less tolerant of vascular changes and even minor haemorrhages or emboli can have considerable effects on overall function (Christiansen and Grzybowski, 1999).

The eye

Structures of the eye

Each eye is located in a deep cavity in the skull called the orbital cavity. The eyeball is a hollow fluid-filled sphere composed of three layers. It is divided into anterior and posterior compartments. Of the total surface area of the eye, only the anterior 1/6th is exposed (Tortora and Derrickson, 2009). The outermost layer is composed of the sclera and cornea. The sclera, which makes up the posterior 5/6th of the eyeball, is composed of white, fibrous tissue. Anteriorly, the sclera is continuous with the cornea in the front of the eye which is transparent. The sclera maintains eye shape and allows the attachment of muscles. There are six muscles that are attached to the sclera by small tendons, these muscles control eye movement. The cornea is convex in shape and is involved in refracting (bending) light to bring it into focus at the back of the eyeball.

The choroid lines the posterior 5/6th of the inner surface of the sclera (Waugh and Grant, 2006). The choroid contains a large amount of melanin and thus appears black. This black pigmentation absorbs stray light rays so that light is not reflected inside the eye (Seeley et al., 2005). The choroid contains many blood vessels that nourish the retina.

The choroid terminates at a structure called the ciliary body. The ciliary body contains smooth muscles (and is therefore not under conscious control). The lens is suspended from these muscles by suspensory ligaments which protrude from this body. The lens is a transparent, flexible, biconvex disc. By contracting and relaxing these muscles, it is possible to change the shape of the lens and thus ensure light rays are brought to a focus on a point at the back of the eye in the central fovea. This area contains only cone cells; cones are the nerve cells responsible for detecting colour.

The iris is the coloured portion of the eye. It is composed of circular and longitudinal muscles. The iris is attached to the anterior edge of the ciliary body and sits in front of the lens. The iris determines how much light enters the eye. Its diameter is controlled by autonomic reflexes via the 3rd cranial (oculomotor) nerve. The activity of the iris protects the sensitive retina from excessive, harmful light rays.

The retina is the vascular innermost lining of the eye where the light-sensitive nerve cells, rods and cones, are found. Cones are responsible for colour vision and function predominantly in daytime. The rods are most active in night vision.

Aqueous humour and vitreous humour

The anterior compartment that lies between the cornea and the front of the lens contain a fluid known as aqueous humour. This compartment is divided into two chambers. The anterior chamber lies between the cornea and the front of the iris. The posterior chamber lies behind the iris but in front of the lens. This is a fluid which maintains the eye's shape. There is a continuous circulation of aqueous humour, such that it is completely replaced every 90 minutes (Tortora and Derrickson, 2009). Vitreous humour is found in the posterior compartment between the lens and the retina. This jelly-like substance prevents the eye from collapsing.

Accessory structures

The accessory structures of the eye consist of eyebrows, eyelids, lacrimal (tear) apparatus and eyelashes. All have protective functions. They prevent dust, sweat and foreign objects from entering the eye. Tears are formed in lacrimal glands; they keep the eye moist, the tears then flow into the nose via the nasolacrimal ducts located at the inner aspect of the eye.

Physiology of vision

In order to see clearly, light must be brought into focus on the retina. This is achieved through a number of mechanisms and these are discussed below.

Refraction

Refraction refers to how light waves are bent as they move from one medium to another. Moving through the different structures in the eye, the light rays bend four times. The result of all this bending is that the light rays land on a portion of the retina which is rich in nerve endings.

Accommodation

To ensure that large objects and small objects can both be projected on the back of the eye, it is necessary to have a mechanism in the eye which can alter its capacity to bend waves. The lens of the eye does this. It can become fat and squat and thus bends waves acutely or can become flat and thin thus hardly bending them at all. This manipulation of waves is called accommodation.

Constriction

The pupil is an open space which allows light to enter the eye. It is created by the iris which is composed of circular and radial muscles. By contracting or relaxing, the iris widens or reduces the hole through which light enters the eye. Thus, the entry of light into the eye is controlled and we are not blinded in bright light and we can see reasonably well in dark conditions.

Convergence

As we have two eyes, it is important that light from an image strikes the same area in each retina. In this way a clear image will be produced. To achieve this, the eyes will move, or converge, to bring the object into a clear focus. Convergence is controlled by the ANS activating the external muscles of the eye. If this did not occur, the two eyes would focus on slightly different parts of an object resulting in double vision or diplopia.

Retina and the conversion of light to an electrical signal

The retina is the photosensitive portion of the eye, that is, it is sensitive to light. When light hits the rods and cones within the retina, photosensitive pigments within them break-down and action potentials are generated. The action potentials are carried via the optic nerve (second cranial nerve) through the thalamus to the visual cortex in the occipital lobe of the brain where they are interpreted. It should be noted (Figure 4.2) that the information from half of each image is carried to the opposite side of the brain.

Visual purple (rhodopsin) is a photosensitive pigment which is only found in rods. This pigment requires an adequate supply of vitamin A for proper functioning. If lacking in vitamin A, a person may suffer from night blindness in which they have difficulty in seeing in dim light. The cones contain different photosensitive pigments that are sensitive to coloured light, namely red, green and blue. We can see a wide range of colours as cones are stimulated in different combinations.

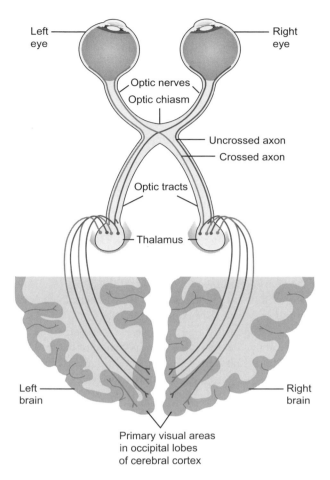

Figure 4.2 Diagram of visual pathways. (Reproduced from Tortora and Derrickson (2007). With permission from John Wiley & Sons.)

Ageing changes in the eye

The hairs on the eyebrow and eyelashes lose melanin and become grey while the skin around the eyelids loosen and wrinkle. The muscles of the eyelids lose tone and elasticity. There is loss of orbital fat resulting in the eyes sinking deeper into the orbit. This limits an individual's upward gaze (Roach, 2001).

The cornea also alters with ageing. It becomes flatter, thicker and loses its smooth appearance. These changes give the cornea a dull, less transparent appearance and increase the risk of astigmatism (Heath and Schofield, 1999). The cornea loses endothelial cells which lessens corneal sensitivity. This reduces awareness of any eye injury. Epithelial cells within the cornea also decrease in number (Roach, 2001).

The iris becomes paler due to the loss of black pigment giving the iris a washed-out appearance. The arcus senilis, which is thought to be an accumulation of lipids, surrounds the periphery of the iris either partially or fully and resembles a milky or grey ring. The size of the pupil reduces by the age of 60 so that it is 2/3 of the size of a younger adult's pupil. The smaller pupil reduces the amount of light reaching the retina, thus contributing to a loss in visual acuity (Roach, 2001). The reduction in visual acuity due to a change in pupil size has more significance at night as greater time is required to adapt to diminishing light levels and darkness.

The depth of the anterior chamber of the eye decreases as the lens thickens. Less aqueous humour is secreted from the ciliary body but as there is an overall reduction in outflow of fluid from anterior and posterior chambers the intraocular pressure remains within normal limits (Roach, 2001). The sclera may become yellow so that opacity is lost and stray light can now enter the eye, thus reducing visual acuity.

The lens becomes larger, thicker, stiffer and denser due to the ageing process. The lens also loses elasticity. The change in the size of the lens is thought to be caused by either biochemical changes in the nucleus and the capsule (Heath and Schofield, 1999) or because debris from cells collect in the capsule (Roach, 2001). The lens becomes yellow and darkens so that colour perception changes. Colour clarity reduces by 25% in the fifties and by 70% in the sixties (Heath and Schofield, 1999). Loss of elasticity in the lens results in a reduced ability to focus known as presbyopia. This can be corrected by wearing bifocal glasses or convex lenses (Lueckenotte, 2000).

Ageing changes in the suspensory ligaments, ciliary muscles and parasympathetic nerve supply to the iris lead to a decrease in accommodation of the lens. The ciliary muscle reduces in length and loses elasticity. Connective tissue replaces muscle tissue which reduces the ability of the lens to change shape in order to accommodate and focus clearly on objects which are nearby.

The vitreous humour becomes thinner and loses some of its fluid with age (Meisami et al., 2003). This results in the production of harmless floaters (small particles of debris that 'float' in the vitreous humour) appearing in the visual field. Occlusions in the arterial and venous retinal blood vessels occur, leading to loss of some of the cells in the retinal and optic pathways. These losses reduce the ability to see detail, contrast and colour. The thinning of the vitreous humour, the yellowing of the lens, the increasingly smaller pupil and the presence of floaters all contribute to a reduction in peripheral vision which limits the size of the visual field, reduces night vision and impairs depth perception in the older adult. Glare sensitivity also occurs, which is a reduction in visual acuity in bright light and is thought to be related to the lens scattering light (Heath and Schofield, 1999).

The ear

Normal structure and function

In order to perceive sound, it is necessary to collect sound waves from the external environment and convert them into an electrical signal which is then interpreted within the auditory areas in the right and left temporal lobe of the cerebrum (Figure 4.3).

Sound waves reach the ear via the external auditory canal. This consists of the pinna or outer ear and the canal itself. The canal is ~2.5-cm long and slightly S-shaped. It is lined

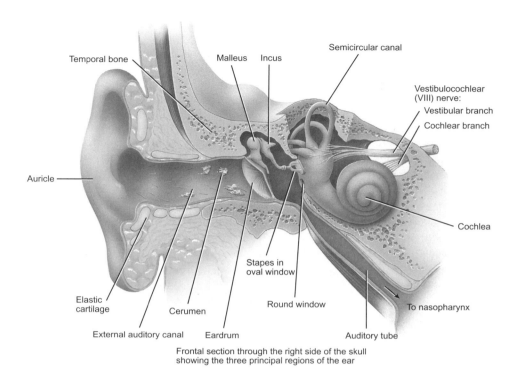

Temporal bone

Malleus　Incus

Semicircular canal

Vestibulocochlear
(VIII) nerve:

Vestibular branch

Cochlear branch

Auricle

Cochlea

Stapes in
oval window

Elastic
cartilage

Cerumen

Round window

To nasopharynx

External auditory canal　Eardrum

Auditory tube

Frontal section through the right side of the skull
showing the three principal regions of the ear

Figure 4.3　Diagram of ear. (Reproduced from Tortora and Derrickson (2007). With permission from John Wiley & Sons.)

with small hairs and ceruminous glands. These glands produce cerumen (earwax) that helps trap dust and other foreign objects, thus protecting the tympanic membrane.

The ear is composed of three compartments: the outer ear, the middle ear and the inner ear. The tympanic membrane (eardrum) separates the outer ear from the middle ear. This membrane is a thin membrane of connective tissue sandwiched between an inner and outer layer. The outer layer is composed of hairless skin and is continuous with the ear canal. The inner layer is composed of mucous membrane and is continuous with the lining of the middle ear (Waugh and Grant, 2006).

The middle ear is a small air-filled cavity which contains the three auditory ossicles (small bones), namely the malleus, incus and stapes. Two covered openings are found on the inner aspect of the middle ear which connects it with the inner ear. These are the round and oval windows. These are small membrane-covered openings in the inner ear. The stapes is attached to the membrane of the oval window. A tube originates in the anterior portion of the middle ear that connects with the nasopharynx. This is known as the pharyngotympanic or Eustachian tube (Tortora and Derrickson, 2009). During swallowing and yawning, the tube opens allowing for the equalisation of air pressure on either side of the tympanic membrane.

The stapes connects to the oval window of the inner ear. The inner ear is a cavity within the temporal bone on each side of the skull. It is composed of an outer bony labyrinth that encloses an inner membranous labyrinth. The bony labyrinth consists of:

- The vestibule
- The cochlea
- Three semicircular canals.

The space between the outer bony labyrinth and the inner membranous labyrinth is filled with a fluid known as perilymph. The space within the inner membranous labyrinth is filled with endolymph.

The vestibule lies nearest to the middle ear and contains the oval and round windows. The cochlea resembles a snail's shell in appearance (Waugh and Grant, 2006). The cochlea contains the organ of Corti which is the organ of hearing. It is within the cochlea, through the action of specialised hair cells, that the sound energy is converted to an electrical signal which is then conveyed via the auditory nerve (8th cranial nerve) to the respective temporal lobe of the cerebrum where the sound is perceived and interpreted.

The semicircular canals are a set of three tubes arranged in different planes and are continuous with the vestibule. The semicircular canals and the vestibule contain specialised hair cells and are concerned with posture and balance rather than hearing.

Physiology of sound

Sound waves are concentrated and carried down the external auditory canal causing vibration in the tympanic membrane. The movement of the membrane is transmitted through the bony ossicles. The ossicles amplify the vibration of the tympanic membrane up to 20-fold, causing an inward and outward movement of the oval window of the cochlea. Two muscles attached to the malleus and stapes can limit their movement when loud noise threatens to damage the inner ear (Seeley et al., 2005).

Perilymph and endolymph

Vibration of the oval window sets the perilymph in the scala vestibuli and scala tympani in motion. This creates a 'ripple' of energy that causes bowing of the scala media. In this way the sound energy is transmitted to the endolymph which is set in motion.

The organ of Corti

The organ of Corti lies on the basilar membrane. It consists of fine hair-like protrusions. The hairs are roofed by the jelly-like tentorial membrane. Movement of the endolymph moves the tentorial membrane which in turn pulls the hair-like protrusions. These hairs are actually protrusions from cell bodies. Their movement provokes action potentials in the cells. The impulses generated are conducted to the temporal lobe via the 8th cranial nerve. The hair-like protrusions can be likened to the keys on a piano, the high keys being nearest to the oval window, and the movement of the endolymph determines which keys are 'pressed'.

Ageing changes in hearing and vestibular function

Hearing loss is common but not inevitable with advancing age. However, 50% of people over 75 experience hearing difficulties (Lueckenotte, 2000). Presbycusis describes hearing loss due to age-related sensori-neural changes. Hearing loss is thought to be as a result of loss of hair cells and nerve fibres within the organ of Corti near the oval window, where high-pitched sound is converted to nerve impulses. Hearing loss is more noticeable in relation to high-pitched sounds and consonants which are difficult to hear correctly (Lueckenotte, 2000).

The process is bilateral and starts from the age of 40. Hearing is not as accurate when there are high levels of background noise. Loss of hearing acuity makes it more challenging to identify direction of sounds. This can make it problematic for older adults in company, where they may have difficulty in detecting the direction of speech.

The atrophy of the sebaceous and apocrine glands makes the cerumen drier. The external auditory canal narrows and the hairs within it become course and stiffer. These changes can lead to impaction of cerumen. Excessive wax accumulation in the ear will exaggerate presbycusis.

Otosclerosis or arthritic conditions affect the joints between the malleus and the stapes. This reduces vibration of these bones, resulting in conductive hearing loss. The vestibular system demonstrates some degeneration associated with ageing. Cell loss occurs in both the vestibule and semicircular canals which are involved in detecting movement, position and acceleration of the head. These changes are brought about by decreases in both hair cell receptors in the vestibule and semicircular canals and nerve fibres in the 8th cranial nerve.

Conditions associated with communication difficulty in older adults

In the following section we shall examine a number of conditions that, if present in older people, may cause difficulties in communicating effectively.

Delirium

Delirium is a transient organic mental syndrome which is typified by a reduction in level of consciousness, a reduced capacity to focus on tasks in hand, perceptual disturbances and memory impairment (American Psychiatric Association, 2000).

Patients over the age of 65 are at higher risk of developing delirium when hospitalised when compared to those under the age of 65 (McCusker et al., 2001). However, older adults can also be admitted to hospital *with* delirium if they have, for example, an underlying infection. In fact, the presence of delirium in such patients may be the presenting feature of the infection. Incidence of delirium development in older adults who are hospitalised ranges from 15% (Rudberg et al., 1997) to 65% (Inouye et al., 1999). Delirium is one of the commonest post-operative complications in older adults, which occurs in 15–25% of older people following elective surgery and 25–65% of older people following emergency admission and surgery (Marcantonio et al., 2000).

Table 4.2   Common symptoms of delirium.

Fluctuating levels of consciousness
Fluctuating levels of awareness
Disorientation to time, person and place
Impaired mental function
Memory lapses
Poor attention span
Illusions
Hallucinations especially visual
Delusions which are often persecutory
Aggressive behaviour
Disturbances of sleep–wake cycle

As part of the ageing process, there is a reduction in the number of neurones, a reduction in brain neurotransmitters such as gamma aminobutyric acid (GABA) and acetylcholine (Ach) and a reduction in cerebral blood flow (Adams et al., 1997). Associated with these normal ageing changes is a decline in the physiologic reserve that enables the brain to cope with the stress of metabolic disturbances or infections. As a result of this decline, it may be that responses to stressors are less effective in old age. This may make the older adult more susceptible to the development of delirium under stressful conditions whether they are physical, psychological or environmental (Farley and McLafferty, 2007).

Delirium develops fairly rapidly from a matter of hours to a few days. Symptoms are varied but are generally worse during the night (Table 4.2).

The risk factors for delirium are many and varied. The following list identifies some common predisposing factors for the development of delirium:

- Old age
- Underlying infection
- Sensory deprivation
- Sensory impairments
- Medical illness
- Pain
- Prescribed drugs including antipsychotic and narcotic drugs
- Hypoxaemia
- Emergency admission to hospital
- Being moved to a new environment
- Use of physical restraints including bed rails
- Urinary catheterisation
- Dehydration
- Environmental factors
- Dementia
- Depression

- Alcohol overuse
- Abnormal urea, electrolytes and blood glucose levels
- Malnutrition
- Social isolation
- Surgery.

There are three different types of delirium: hyperactive, which is detected by many health-care staff; hypoactive, which goes largely undetected by health-care staff and a mixed delirium, where the person expresses symptoms of both hyper- and hypoactive delirium. Hypoactive delirium is more common than the more readily recognised hyperactive type and includes the features of under-activity, apathy and lethargy. Features of hyperactive delirium include being over alert, increased psychomotor activity and a heightened response to all stimuli.

Assessment for delirium

The mini-mental state examination – MMSE (Folstein et al., 1975) is a commonly used assessment tool to help identify cognitive changes in older adults and as such is frequently used in delirium. It measures a person's cognitive function and takes around 10 minutes to complete.

The MMSE measures are:

- Orientation
- Registration
- Attention
- Calculation
- Recall
- Language ability.

and can be used to identify baseline measurements as well as cognitive changes over time. However, the MMSE was not specifically designed for use in delirium, but Rapp et al. (2000) state it is nevertheless a useful tool when assessing mental status. However, patients must be able to see and communicate both verbally and in writing in order to respond to this tool.

The Confusion Assessment Method (CAM) tool assesses 10 symptoms of delirium and is recommended by the Royal College of Physicians (2006). The whole assessment can be completed in less than 5 minutes. The symptoms assessed are:

- The acuteness of onset
- Fluctuating course where the effects of delirium peak and trough
- Inattention
- Disorganised thinking
- Altered levels of consciousness
- Disorientation
- Memory impairment
- Perceptual disturbances

- Psychomotor activity
- Sleep–wake disturbance.

Although this assessment involves the use of a structured instrument, users may be required to make some subjective clinical judgements during the assessment (Rapp et al., 2000).

Management

Following a diagnosis of delirium, several nursing strategies can be utilised to minimise the impact this temporary condition may have on the individual and their carers.

In 40% of older adults who become delirious, their medications are directly implicated in this development. As a result of this, prescribed pharmacological agents should be considered as a factor in the development of delirium (Brown and Boyle, 2002). It is not just individual drugs and drug interactions which should be reviewed here. The prescribing physician or pharmacist should also note if new drugs have been prescribed recently and, if so, how many different drugs have been prescribed. According to Kaplan et al. (2003), patients who receive more than three new medications together are at increased risk of developing delirium.

The presence of infection is a well-documented precipitating factor for dementia (Schor et al., 1992). Health-care professionals have to recognise that older adults are at risk of opportunistic infections as their immune systems are not as effective as compared to younger adults. Health-care professionals should also be aware that infection may not present 'typically' in older adults. Confusion may be the initial presenting feature of infection rather than any other typical sign or symptom of commonly associated infection (McLafferty and Farley, 2007). If the presence of confusion is linked to the possibility of infection, health-care professionals can further assess the presence or absence of infection and initiate early treatment as required. This proactive approach to management and care can reduce the risk of delirium or may actually prevent delirium from occurring.

Pain and management of pain have been implicated in the development of delirium (Schuurmans et al., 2001). A pain assessment (see pages 54–59) should therefore be carried out, appropriate analgesia administered and its effectiveness or otherwise noted during an evaluation of its effects. Any analgesia known to contribute to confusion should be avoided.

Health-care professionals should also be aware of the possible effects environmental factors can have on a person's cognitive functions. Brown and Boyle (2002) suggest that environmental factors, and being moved to a new environment, can contribute to delirium. Older adults are not only at risk from development of delirium following admission to hospital, they are also at risk if they are temporarily moved (boarded out) to another clinical environment. This should therefore be avoided in older adults when it is necessary to temporarily 'board' patients because of pressure on beds.

Noise levels should be kept to a minimum at all times and patient areas should be well lit (Potter, 2004). Night lights should be used where appropriate to reduce the risk of patients misinterpreting the environment and objects within it. Cues can be provided to orientate people to time, person and place. Such cues can include photographs, pictures, clocks, calendars and signs above different areas within the environment (Agostini et al., 2001).

The initial nursing assessment should include measures to detect sensory or perceptual deficit (Parikh and Chung, 1995). Visual and hearing tests should be conducted regularly and cerumen removal carried out if necessary. Sensory impairment can be reduced by ensuring that visual and hearing aids are available, working and used.

The use of physical restraints such as bed rails and chair tables may precipitate delirium (Inouye and Charpentier, 1996). Therefore, the use of physical restraints should be limited and if used need to be fully justified. Potter (2004) goes further and states they should only be used when patients are at risk of harming themselves and only following a full risk assessment.

In management of patients, the presence of relatives is often undervalued. In relation to delirium, Meagher (2001) describes the importance of the presence of relatives as they heighten the patient's feelings of security and orientation. Indeed, the presence of relatives may not only help with orientation but their presence can also assist with the reorientation process. Health-care professionals should therefore welcome and encourage family members and friends to visit and interact with the patient. This not only provides support for the individual but also helps maintain continuity with life outside the inpatient setting (Schofield, 2002).

Pain in older people

Pain is described as a multidimensional experience that is unique to each individual (Royal College of Physicians, 2007). It can interfere with a person's physical, psychosocial and spiritual well-being.

Pain afflicts the daily life of many older people, but it is not a normal component of the ageing process although older people and sometimes health professionals think it is. It is often accepted as an inevitable consequence of ageing (Bird, 2005). The experience of pain which is common among older people is often ignored by policy makers and service planners (Royal College of Physicians, 2007).

Pain limits functional ability and severely impairs an older person's quality of life (Jakobsson et al., 2007). Sometimes there are difficulties for older people in articulating their pain, especially if they have disorders including dementia, some forms of stroke and PD (Royal College of Physicians, 2007). Therefore, the assessment and management of pain in older people requires excellent verbal and observational skills. Nurses must be able to use observation in order to recognise the non-verbal manifestations of pain. Acute pain will be experienced by older people, but the main problem is chronic pain which is experienced by a reasonable number of older people usually as a result of a long-term condition such as arthritis, osteoporosis or stroke. The effects of pain for older people are wide ranging. As mobility can be limited, there may be an increasing reluctance to take part in activities both of which can lead to depressed mood (Jakobsson et al., 2007).

Epidemiology of pain for older people

Pain is experienced by 49–83% of older people (Epps, 2001). The percentages are so variable because writers use differing parameters when they study pain, making it difficult to identify the scale of the problem in older people. However, 66% of older people believe that their pain will not be taken seriously which is not surprising when so many older people are told that it is 'just their age'. As there is an expectation of pain in older age, it is not surprising that 40% of older people do not truly understand the consequences of untreated pain (Brockopp et al., 1996). Older people receive less analgesia than younger people (Morrison and Sui, 2000). People with dementia receive less analgesia than older people without dementia (about three times less likely to receive analgesia) (Morrison and Siu, 2000). Interestingly, 53% of patients do not understand the benefits of taking regular analgesia (Brockopp et al., 1996).

Many older people are reluctant to consult health professionals so they are resigned to bearing pain, ambivalent about treatment and reluctant to express pain.

The consequences of poor pain management include depression, poor concentration, fatigue and memory impairment. Physical effects in relation to the poor management of pain include a reduction in mobility, decreased functional ability, disturbed sleep, decreased social activities, increased isolation and decreased appetite.

Pain assessment is a value-laden method by which health-care workers interpret the patient's pain (Marvin, 1995). There are a number of pain assessment tools that can be used which fall into two main categories. Tools that are one-dimensional and tools that are multidimensional. Uni-dimensional tools measure pain intensity while multidimensional tools take a more holistic approach by including the patient's experience (Bird, 2005). Therefore, other issues should be included in pain assessment and they are pain affect and pain location. Pain affect includes how the patient feels about their pain and the emotions that the patient attaches to the pain, while pain location should include the origin and radiation of the pain and whether it is acute or chronic (Jensen and Karoly, 1992). An assessment of pain should routinely be done using a standardised intensity rating scale.

Criteria for choosing a pain assessment tool

- Is it valid and reliable?
- Is it appropriate for the client group?
- Is it easily and quickly understood?
- Is it patient and client friendly?
- Is it easily scored and recorded?
- Is it comprehensive?
- Is it readily available for use?
- Is it inexpensive?

Available pain assessment scales include:

- Numerical scales
- Visual analogue scales (VASs)
- Verbal rating scales
- Faces pain scale
- McGill pain questionnaire (MPQ).

No pain								Worst pain imaginable		
0	1	2	3	4	5	6	7	8	9	10

Figure 4.4   An example of an NRS.

No	Mild	Moderate	Severe	Very severe
Pain	Pain	Pain	Pain	Pain

Figure 4.5   An example of a verbal rating scale.

Numerical rating scales (NRSs) normally have an 11-point continuum from 0 to 10. The patient is asked to rate their pain, where 0 is no pain and 10 is the worst pain imaginable. Verbal administration of the NRS can be used if patients have either physical or visual impairments. People may also have difficulty applying numbers to their pain (Bird, 2005). Figure 4.4 shows an example of an NRS.

Verbal rating scales (Figure 4.5) have 4–6 descriptors of pain, for example very severe, severe, moderate, mild, none. It is therefore the patient's responsibility to interpret the words making it less sensitive than other scales (Briggs, 2003).

Verbal rating/descriptor and NRSs best quantify the intensity of pain in older people with no cognitive impairment and those with mild to moderate cognitive impairment. In other words, they give good reliability and validity for rating pain in older people (Royal College of Physicians, 2007).

The faces pain scale was originally designed to be used for children, but it has been used with older adults. This scale should be considered when nurses suspect the accuracy of pain measurement is affected by fatigue, or low physical or mental state, if there is a problem with being able to read or language barriers are evident. However, the faces scale is less effective than the NRSs and verbal rating scales (Stuppy, 1998). Cognitively intact older adults can use the faces pain scale with good test–retest reproducibility; however, when they are asked to place the faces in the correct order of pain intensity older people cannot always do so. This therefore raises serious doubts about the validity of the faces scale.

The VAS has a 10-cm line with anchors of no pain and worst pain at each end of the line (Figure 4.6). The patient marks on the line to indicate how intense their pain is. If this scale is to be used in older people, then health professionals will need to consider the size of the print which should be large enough to make it easy for patients to see. The surface should be checked for glare as any reflections will reduce visibility and clarity. The patient has to make their own mark on the scale. This should not be done by the nurse (Bird, 2005). Of all the scales, the VASs are the least effective. Older people may have both physical and conceptual difficulties in using VASs, resulting in a significant failure rate for this scale when used by older adults.

The MPQ is an example of a multidimensional assessment tool. However, the verbal descriptors were developed by a group of psychology students. Therefore, its use as a pain assessment tool has been questioned. Nevertheless, Gagliese et al. (1999) have commented that the MPQ may be used either in its long or short format for older people.

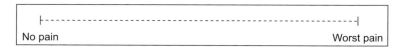

Figure 4.6   An example of a VAS.

There are other available pain assessment tools, but as with other assessment tools, they should be evaluated for use with older people.

However, no matter the scale used, a number of factors must be taken into account when trying to assess older people's pain including the ability to focus, colour discrimination and visual acuity, as they all decline with advancing age.

Pain scales should therefore use large clear letters/numbers preferably with high contrast, that is black and white, they should be non-reflective and they should be presented under good lighting.

Due to a strong correlation between the presence of pain and mood, mood should also be assessed in all older people with pain. The Royal College of Physicians (2007) recommend using either the hospital anxiety and depression scale (HADS) or the geriatric depression scale (GDS).

It has already been identified that some of the scales above can be used for people with mild to moderate cognitive impairment; however, there are now specific pain scales for patients who may be unable to articulate their pain due to a disorder causing cognitive impairment, the most common disorder being dementia. Patients with dementia may not respond quickly to pain assessments so patience is very important. However, there are problems with these scales as validity and reliability data are limited or unavailable for many of the instruments.

Observation and clinical judgement are particularly important in patients who are unable to verbalise their pain if they have difficulty communicating or have cognitive deficits. People with moderate deficits are still able to reliably indicate that they are in pain and therefore should be believed. Observations should include facial expressions, body movements, verbalisations, vocalisations, physiology and changes in interpersonal interactions, changes in activity levels and patterns. It is also important to involve relatives and families as they know the person better and are able to help the nurse identify when a patient is in pain or how the pain manifests itself in the patient.

The Abbey pain scale (Figure 4.7) is used for measuring pain in people with dementia who have difficulties verbalising words. It is a one-page assessment tool that uses non-verbal observable cues and then scores observations to establish what level of pain the person is experiencing.

The scale can be used both as an assessment tool before a pain intervention and afterwards as a measure of effectiveness and success of the intervention.

 Point for Practice

Consider your client/patient group. Evaluate your current pain assessment tools and in light of what you have learned reflect upon their suitability.

The Abbey Pain Scale
For measurement of pain in people with dementia who cannot verbalise

How to use scale: While observing the resident, score questions 1 to 6.

Name of resident: ....

Name and designation of person completing the scale: ....

Date: ....Time: ....

Latest pain relief given was…………………..… at ....hrs.

Q1. **Vocalisation**
    e.g. whimpering, groaning, crying   Q1 ☐
    Absent 0   *Mild 1*   *Moderate 2*   *Severe 3*

Q2. **Facial expression**
    e.g. looking tense, frowning, grimacing, looking frightened   Q2 ☐
    Absent 0   *Mild 1*   *Moderate 2*   *Severe 3*

Q3. **Change in body language**
    e.g. fidgeting, rocking, guarding part of body, withdrawn   Q3 ☐
    Absent 0   *Mild 1*   *Moderate 2*   *Severe 3*

Q4. **Behavioural change**
    e.g. increased confusion, refusing to eat, alteration in usual patterns   Q4 ☐
    Absent 0   *Mild 1*   *Moderate 2*   *Severe 3*

Q5. **Physiological change**
    e.g. temperature, pulse or blood pressure outside normal limits, perspiring, flushing or pallor
    Absent 0   *Mild 1*   *Moderate 2*   *Severe 3*   Q5 ☐

Q6. **Physical changes**
    e.g. skin tears, pressure areas, arthritis, contractures, previous injuries   Q6 ☐
    Absent 0   *Mild 1*   *Moderate 2*   *Severe 3*

Add scores for Q1 to Q6 and record here   ⟹   Total pain score   ☐

Now tick the box that matches
the total pain score   ⟹

0–2 No pain	3–7 Mild	8–13 Moderate	14+ Severe

Finally, tick the box which matches
the type of pain   ⟹

Chronic	Acute	Acute on chronic

Abbey J, De Bellis A, Piller N, Esterman A, Giles L, Parker D, Lowcay B. The Abbey Pain Scale. Funded by the JH & JD Gunn Medical Research Foundation 1998–2002.

Figure 4.7   The Abbey pain scale.

Other factors should be included in the assessment.

Nursing assessment has to recognise that older people are often reluctant to acknowledge and report pain so patience and persistence may be required in order to make an accurate pain assessment. Older people do not always use the word pain nor do they apply the word to themselves. Therefore, they may use a wide range of alternative descriptors other than pain itself, which may not be easily recognised by the nurse, to describe their pain. Patients may respond to words such as aching or soreness but do not respond to the word pain. How patients describe their pain may indicate the cause and appropriate treatment. Noting the language that the patient uses to describe their pain on first assessment will assist in subsequent assessment. Pain assessment should be completed as often as necessary and this may vary from patient to patient.

Other factors

- Type or quality of the pain
- Duration of the pain
- Factors that relieve or aggravate pain. For example, does bowel movement relieve the pain or does a meal aggravate the pain?
- Effects of pain on function. Does the pain limit mobility?
- Assessment of cognitive function. Is the patient able to make an evaluation of their pain status?
- Evaluation of social support. Who is at home to care for the patient?
- Cultural environment.

(Adapted from Bird, 2005)

Ineffective treatment of pain has a number of consequences which makes it so important to assess and manage pain appropriately. Ineffective treatment can lead to:

- Decreased quality of life
- Depression
- Anxiety
- Decreased socialisation
- Sleep disturbance
- Decreased mobility
- Under-nutrition.

There are barriers to effective management of pain in older people. It has already been identified that pain is viewed by many as a natural occurrence in old age. This may lead to under reporting of pain, it can prevent accurate assessment as if the patient does not report pain, they probably will not be assessed for pain. Older people may therefore be denied pain relief measures.

Older people may feel that they should be stoical about pain and this may be directly linked to the stiff upper lip attitude that has been fairly prevalent in older generations within the United Kingdom. There is a perception that older people do not feel pain as much as younger people; however, pain intensity and frequency increase with age. Older people may fear the meaning of the pain, they may worry about the pain being linked to a serious medical condition such as cancer and as a result may not present themselves for diagnostic investigation (Gloth, 2000). Older people may be fearful that if given strong pain relief they may be at risk of drug addiction. This fear may reduce the likelihood of asking for or complying with prescribed medications for pain relief.

Management of pain for older people

Pain-relieving strategies will include the use of prescribed and non-prescribed analgesia. There is a wide range of analgesia that can be used both safely and effectively for older people. It is important that nurses follow protocols when administering analgesia. An individualised approach to the prescription of analgesia is important in order to ensure that older patients are prescribed the most appropriate medications for their pain. It may be necessary to contend with older people's misconceptions about medications. Pain medications should be prescribed at regular intervals as opposed to prescribing them as needed or required. It is also important that nurses use the correct language when trying to ascertain whether older people are in pain.

There are a wide range of non-pharmacological strategies that can also be used in the management of pain which should be considered either as an accompaniment to conventional medications management or as an alternative strategy.

These include:

- Application of heat or cold to the affected area
- Deep breathing exercises
- Distraction including television or reading
- Structured relaxation techniques
- Guided imagery
- Music therapy
- Hypnotherapy
- Transcutaneous electrical nerve stimulation (TENS)
- Reflexology
- Aromatherapy.

(Adapted from Brown, 2004)

Parkinson's disease

Parkinson's disease (PD) is a degenerative disorder of the neurones involved in motor control. It occurs in ~1 person in 100 over the age of 60 (Smith, 2003), although this can vary as there is a higher incidence in rural communities which is thought to be linked to herbicides and pesticides. Heavy metals such as manganese have also been implicated in the development of PD. It occurs more commonly in people over 65 although it does occur in 1 in every 250 people under 65 (Noble, 2007). The evidence is uncertain regarding a genetic link. Currently, there is no known cure for PD. The disease is progressive and can affect movement, mood, cognition, swallowing and communication (Noble, 2007).

The nature and severity of the symptoms and pattern of symptom progression vary from individual to individual.

Pathophysiology

The degeneration of the neurones occurs predominantly in the region of the midbrain called the substantia nigra. The brain cells of the substantia nigra communicate with another part of the brain called the striatum through the neurotransmitter dopamine. Approximately 400 000 special neurones produce dopamine which is required by the brain for signalling the body in relation to proper control of skeletal muscle and coordination. PD occurs when these special neurones are slowly destroyed resulting in a reduction in the production of dopamine leading to a disorganisation of motor signals. The presence of dopamine is vital for the control of voluntary and involuntary movement (Noble, 2007). However, 70% of dopamine production is destroyed before the major signs and symptoms of PD occur (Smith, 2003). PD can be primary or secondary. In primary PD, Lewy bodies, which are abnormal collections of proteins, are found in cells that are dying although they are not present in all cases. Secondary PD is thought to be caused by encephalitis, carbon monoxide poisoning, stroke or metabolic and degenerative disorders.

There are a number of signs and symptoms that appear to be a precursor of the florid symptoms of PD. These include a loss of sense of smell, sleep disorders and constipation (Noble, 2007). Indeed, there may be symptoms of rapid eye movement (REM) sleep behaviour disorder for many years prior to the development of major signs and symptoms of PD (Wolkove et al., 2007). Remember that REM sleep is deep sleep and is the stage where dreams occur. The partner will describe overnight behaviour of the person with PD as being extremely active with the person exhibiting signs of agitation and aggressive behaviour while sleeping (Noble, 2007). Dreams and nightmares may also be associated with prescribed medications to control PD.

In the early stages of PD, signs and symptoms of fatigue, occasional muscle stiffness, handwriting changes or an infrequent tremor of the finger may be present (Wolkove et al., 2007). Other early symptoms experienced by patients include changes in bowel habit leading to increased risk of constipation, sluggish urinary bladder, sexual dysfunction and visual problems. These symptoms are slow and insidious, but they may become more overt as the disease progresses. It should be noted that this is a progressive and unremitting disease.

The clinical features of PD include:

- Symptoms may occur unilaterally at onset and affect coordination.
- Tremors of the fingers at rest which disappear with movement and is described as pill rolling.
- Tremors may also affect the leg or the tongue or one side of the body. Tremors are not present in up to 20% of patients diagnosed with PD; however, it is the first symptom in 75% of cases (Clarke, 2001).
- Muscular rigidity and bradykinesia which is described as slowness of movement. Stiff muscles lead to this slow movement.
- Delay in spontaneity may be present.

- Difficulties with manual dexterity making, for example fastening buttons becomes difficult or tying shoelaces becomes a challenge.
- Delay in initiating gait and movement.
- Altered gait patterns demonstrated by a slow shuffling gait with a noticeable lack of arm swinging. The patient with PD can freeze (sudden stoppage of movement) without warning putting themselves at risk of falling.
- Increased muscle tone described as lead pipe and cog wheel movements.
- Painful muscles and joints with cramps.
- Difficulty in moving or turning in bed.
- Postural instability can cause loss of coordination and balance as demonstrated by clumsy movement.
- Stooped posture.
- Blank facial expression.
- Quiet monotonous speech.
- Takes longer to complete usual daily tasks.

People may also complain of restless legs syndrome which is referred to and defined in Chapter 11 relating to sleeping. Remember, restless legs syndrome is a neurological sensori-motor disorder where the patient complains of tingly and cramping sensations in the legs occurring normally in bed at night leading to an urge to massage the leg in order to obtain relief (Noble, 2007).

Parkinson's disease can also affect the fine muscles that control speech, swallowing and respiration. Therefore, patients may slur their words, stutter, speak in a whisper or a raspy voice or even lose the ability to speak altogether. They may also suffer from difficulties in swallowing which can result in choking and aspiration pneumonia. Difficulties in swallowing may be accompanied by drooling along with loss of ability to seal their lips (Smith, 2003). Bladder problems include features of urinary frequency, urgency and urinary incontinence. Bladder problems occur in more than 66% of patients with PD.

Mental health problems commonly accompany patients with PD. Depression is very common and can impact significantly on quality of life. Anxiety is also very common which can exacerbate the symptoms of PD and initiate a decline in the person's health. This can have a negative impact on a person's rehabilitation and motivation.

Cognitive impairment affects one-third of patients with PD and more than 78% of patients will develop dementia within 8 years from onset of PD. Cognitive impairment can also be present in the early stage of PD and in patients who have not yet been diagnosed with dementia. A number of symptoms are associated with cognitive impairment including a decrease in the ability to process information, difficulties with planning and sequencing where for example, the person with PD may take apart household items then find it very difficult to put them back together again. There may also be a change in personality, poor memory and visual spatial dysfunction. Visual spatial dysfunction is demonstrated when the person has difficulty going through doors or when they find themselves in confined spaces. Behavioural disturbances can occur which are related to the medications used to manage the disease and they may be exhibited through gambling to excess, cravings for food, shopping excessively and hypersexuality (Noble, 2007). As the disease advances, the person may complain of visual hallucinations that frighten themselves and their carers. Finally, psychosis may take the form of visual and tactile hallucinations and delusions.

Diagnosis

Diagnosis is made by a specialist in PD who will take a careful and detailed history from the person and their partner if available. There is no definitive test for PD but blood screening and brain computerised tomography should be completed to rule out other causes such as age-related dementia.

Medical management

If possible medications to control symptoms should be withheld until symptoms appear and become troubling or disabling. This delays the onset of medication side effects and the known effect of 'wearing off' which is described later.

Management of disease is mainly through medications which are aimed at restoring the balance of dopamine as much as possible, providing symptom relief and limiting the distress caused by the symptoms of PD. The mainstay of medications treatment continues to be levodopa which is converted to dopamine once it reaches the brain so that it can produce an anti-parkinsonian effect. For people who are over 60, medication choices may include sustained release levodopa and immediate release levodopa which can be added if sustained release levodopa is not effective in controlling all the symptoms. If maximum levels of prescribed levodopa are reached, a dopamine agonist can then be added.

The effectiveness of pharmacological treatment wears off after ∼3 years of treatment (Snyder and Adler, 2007). This means there is a shortening of the control of symptoms which results in a decrease in the time intervals required between doses. Wearing off can be managed by increasing the frequency of administering levodopa or by the addition of a dopamine agonist or a catechol-*O*-methyltransferase (COMT) inhibitor (Snyder and Adler, 2007). This increases the delivery of levodopa to the brain. However, increasing the frequency and doses of levodopa can induce dyskinesias where there are abnormal involuntary writhing movements. These symptoms are distressing and cause further discomfort to the person.

Other side effects of treatment with dopamine include on/off effects which the person describes as turning off a light switch where they suddenly and unexpectedly change from being mobile to becoming rigid and immobile (Scott, 2002).

There are surgical options for people with PD which include:

- Stereotactic pallidotomy where selective brain tissue is destroyed in the globus pallidus which is a major part of the basal ganglia. This operation improves motor ability leading to an increase in the person's ability to cope with their activities of living, thereby increasing their independence.
- Deep brain stimulation is where electrodes are implanted in the sub thalamic nucleus (also a part of the basal ganglia) to control symptoms. It is most effective in relieving tremor and dyskinesia.
- Implantation of dopamine-producing tissue. This involves the transplantation of foetal cells or stem cells into the basal ganglia of recipients.

Nursing management

Education regarding the signs, symptoms and progress of the disease is very important. Patients need to know that they can maintain a normal lifestyle for many years following diagnosis. Education should also be given in the form of written information which should supplement verbal information given.

As long as the patient is able, they should be encouraged to take part in physical activities including walking, aerobics and muscle strengthening exercises. There are a range of complementary therapies to boost physical and emotional wellness including massage, tai chi, relaxation, visual imagery and music therapy among others.

Regular nutritional assessment is very important. To prevent constipation, a well-balanced diet which is high in fibre should be encouraged. It is also useful to promote a good intake of fluids. Calcium is necessary in order to maintain existing bone structure. Patients with PD may have problems with chewing and swallowing, so a soft, easily swallowed diet should be provided that is high in carbohydrates to replace the calories that are used due to hyperkinesia. Patients may have problems cutting food and this is easily remedied by helping with this at mealtimes. The person with PD may take a long time to eat and drink so they need to be given plenty of time. It may be useful to consider offering small frequent meals.

Listening to the patient is very important as it may be difficult at times to follow and understand what the patient is trying to say. The nurse needs to listen closely to the speech pattern. The patient's voice may be hard to hear. They may mumble or slur their words. The person with PD needs to be given time to answer any questions.

Urinary continence may be improved by using clothing that is straightforward to undo/release. Walking difficulties may be an issue for the person with PD. This can, for example, add to the length of time taken to reach the bathroom. It may therefore be advantageous to have the person seated nearby such facilities.

One of the most difficult aspects for patients with PD is accessing their drugs when they are hospitalised. It can cause a great deal of anxiety resulting in an increase in the symptoms experienced. It is important that patients follow their home medication routine as closely as possible whilst in hospital. If medication routine is altered and patients experience delays in receiving their medications, symptoms of PD can be aggravated. These can include difficulties in communicating and making themselves understood; difficulties in chewing and swallowing food; and an increased risk of falls. Nurses need to follow the patient's normal medication routine and not the routine of the ward medication round (Noble, 2007).

The multidisciplinary team is also vital in the care of patients with PD who should have access to:

- Nurses with a special interest and knowledge of PD
- Occupational therapy for practical help with the activities of living
- Physiotherapy for re-enforcement of motor skills and rehearsal of activity or movement
- A speech and language therapist for speech and swallowing training
- A dietician for ongoing nutritional and dietary advice.

Summary

Communication is a complex activity. Most of the time, we are probably not even aware of the variety of ways and means by which we communicate with one another. However, effective communication is essential, not only to help us meet our basic physiological needs, but so that we can also meet our psychosocial and spiritual needs as well.

Problems of communication can have their foundation in many sources. We may, for example, have problems with sight or hearing. We may have difficulty with our cognitions or our ability to select and form the right words and phrases.

Assessing a client/patient's communication problems requires the health-care professional to be skilled in the selection and use of the appropriate assessment tools. We also need to consider how we approach communication with our clients/patients and whether we could adopt different strategies that would make us more effective communicators.

We have chosen to illustrate the problems that may ensue in this activity of living by examining the effects of delirium, pain and PD on a person's capacity and ability to communicate.

References and further reading

Adams, R.D., Victor, M. and Ropper, A.H. 1997. The neurology of aging. In Adams, R.D., Victor, M. and Ropper, A.H. (Eds). Principles of Neurology. 6th ed. McGraw-Hill, New York, NY, pp. 608–620.

Agostini, J.V., Baker, D.I., Inouye, S.K. and Bogardus, S.T. 2001. Prevention of delirium in older hospitalized patients. In Markowitz, A.J. (Ed). Making Health Care Safer: A Critical Analysis of Patient Safety Practices. Evidence Report/Technology Assessment Number 43. University of California at San Francisco (UCSF)-Stanford University Evidence-based Practice Center, San Francisco, pp. 307–312.

American Psychiatric Association. 2000. Diagnostic and Statistical Manual of Mental Disorders. American Psychiatric Association, Washington, DC.

Bird, J. 2005. Assessing pain in older people. Nursing Standard 19(19), 45–52.

Briggs, E. 2003. The nursing management of pain in older people. Nursing Standard 17(18), 47–53.

Brockopp, D.Y., Warden, S., Colclough, G. and Brockopp, G. 1996. Elderly people's knowledge of and attitude to pain management. British Journal of Nursing 5, 556–562.

Brown, D. 2004. A literature review exploring how health care professionals contribute to the assessment and control of post-operative pain in older people. International Journal of Older People Nursing 13(6b), 74–90.

Brown, T.M. and Boyle, M.F. 2002. Delirium. British Medical Journal 325(7365), 644–647.

Christiansen, J. and Grzybowski, J. 1999. An Introduction to the Biomedical Aspects of Aging. McGraw-Hill, New York, NY.

Clarke, C. 2001. Parkinson's Disease in Practice. RSM Press, London.

Epps, C. 2001. Recognising pain in the institutionalised elder with dementia. Geriatric Nursing 22(2), 71–79.

Farley, A. and McLafferty, E. 2007. Delirium part one: clinical features, risk factors and assessment. Nursing Standard 21(29), 35–40.

Folstein, M.F., Folstein, S. and McHugh, P.R. 1975. "Mini-mental state." A practical method for grading the cognitive state of patients for the clinician. Journal of Psychiatric Research 12(3), 189–198.

Gagliese, L., Katz, J. and Melzack, R. 1999. Pain in the elderly. In Melzack, R. and Wall, P. (Eds). Textbook of Pain. 4th ed. Churchill Livingstone, London.

Gloth, F.M. 2000. Geriatric pain: factors that limit pain relief and increase complications. Geriatrics 55, 46–54.

Heath, H. and Schofield, I. 1999. Healthy Ageing. Nursing Older People. Mosby, London.

Inouye, S.K. and Charpentier, P.A. 1996. Precipitating factors for delirium in hospitalized elderly person: a predictive model and interrelationship with baseline vulnerability. Journal of the American Medical Association 275(1), 852–857.

Inouye, S.K., Schlesinger, M.J. and Lydon, T.J. 1999. Delirium: a symptom of how hospital care is failing older persons and a window to improve quality of hospital care. The American Journal of Medicine 106(5), 565–573.

Jakobsson, U., Halberg, I.R. and Westergren, A. 2007. Exploring determinants for quality of life among older people in pain and in need of help for daily living. Journal of Clinical Nursing 16(3a), 95–104.

Jensen, M. and Karoly, P. 1992. Self-report scales and procedures for assessing pain in adults. In Turk, D. and Melzack, R. (Eds). Handbook of Pain Assessment. Guilford Press, New York, NY.

Kaplan, N.M., Palmer, B.F. and Roche, V. 2003. Etiology and management of delirium. South Western Internal Medicine Conference. The American Journal of the Medical Sciences 325(1), 20–30.

Linton, A. and Matteson, M. 1997. Age-related changes in the neurological system. In Matteson, M., McConnell, E.S. and Linton, A.D. (Eds). Gerontological Nursing: Concepts and Practice. 2nd ed. WB Saunders Company, Philadelphia, PA.

Lueckenotte, A.G. 2000. Gerontologic Nursing. 2nd ed. Mosby, St. Louis, MO.

Marcantonio, E.R., Flacker, J.M., Michaels, M. and Resnick, N.M. 2000. Delirium is independently associated with poor functional recovery after hip fracture. Journal of the American Geriatrics Society 48(6), 618–624.

Marvin, J. 1995. Pain assessment versus measurement. Journal of Burn Care and Rehabilitation 16(3, Part 2), 348–357.

McCusker, J., Cole, M., Dendukuri, N., Belzile, E. and Primeau, F. 2001. Delirium in older medical inpatients and subsequent cognitive and functional status: a prospective study. Canadian Medical Association Journal 165(5), 575–583.

McLafferty, E. and Farley, A. 2007. Delirium part two: nursing management. Nursing Standard 21(30), 42–46.

Meagher, D.J. 2001. Delirium: optimising management (clinical review). British Medical Journal 322(7279), 144–149.

Meisami, E., Brown, C. and Emerle, H. 2003. Sensory systems: normal aging, disorders and treatments of vision and hearing in humans. In Timiras, P. (Ed). Physiological Basis of Aging and Geriatrics. 3rd ed. CRC Press, Boca Raton, FL.

Morrison, R. and Siu, A. 2000. A comparison of pain and its treatment in advanced dementia and cognitively intact patients with hip fracture. Journal of Pain and Symptom Management 19(4), 240–248.

Noble, C. 2007. Understanding Parkinson's disease. Nursing Standard 21(34), 48–56.

Parikh, S.S. and Chung, F. 1995. Postoperative delirium in the elderly. Anesthesia and Analgesia 80(6), 1223–1232.

Potter, J.F. 2004. The older orthopaedic patient: general considerations. Clinical Orthopaedics and Related Research 425, 44–49.

Rapp, C.G., Wakefield, B., Kundrat, M. et al. 2000. Acute confusion assessment instruments: clinical versus research usability. Applied Nursing Research 13(1), 37–45.

Redfern, S.J. and Ross, F.M. 2001. Nursing Older People. 3rd ed. Churchill Livingstone, Edinburgh.

Roach, S. 2001. Introductory Gerontological Nursing. Lippincott, Philadelphia, PA.

Royal College of Physicians. 2006. The Prevention, Diagnosis and Management of Delirium in Older People. Number 6. Concise Guidance to Good Practice. Royal College of Physicians, London.

Royal College of Physicians, British Geriatric Society, British Pain Society. 2007. The Assessment of Pain in Older People: National Guidelines. Concise Guidance to Good Practice Series no. 8. Royal College of Physicians, London.

Rudberg, M.A., Pompei, P., Foreman, M.D., Ross, R.E. and Cassel, C.K. 1997. The natural history of delirium in older hospitalized patients: a syndrome of heterogeneity. Age and Ageing 26(3), 169–174.

Saladin, K.S. 2001. Anatomy and Physiology. 2nd ed. McGraw-Hill, Boston, MA.

Schofield, I. 2002. Assessing for delirium. Nursing Older People 14(7), 31–34.

Schor, J.D., Levkoff, S.E. and Lipsitz, L.A. 1992. Risk factors for delirium in hospitalized elderly. Journal of the American Medical Association 267(6), 827–831.

Schuurmans, M.J., Duursma, S.A. and Shortridge-Baggett, L.M. 2001. Early recognition of delirium: review of the literature. Journal of Clinical Nursing 10(6), 721–729.

Scott, S. 2002. Understanding the challenge of Parkinson's disease. Nursing Standard 16(41), 48–55.

Seeley, R.R., Stephens, T.D. and Tate, P. 2003. Anatomy and Physiology. 6th ed. McGraw-Hill, London.

Seeley, R.R., Stephens, T.D. and Tate, P. 2005. Essentials of Anatomy and Physiology. 5th ed. McGraw-Hill, Boston, MA.

Smith, L.P. 2003. Steady the course of Parkinson's disease. Nursing Management 34(4), 36–40.

Snyder, C.H. and Adler, C.H. 2007. The patient with Parkinson's disease: Part 1 – treating the motor symptoms. Journal of the American Academy of Nurse Practitioners 19, 179–197.

Stuppy, D. 1998. The faces pain scale: reliability and validity with mature adults. Applied Nursing Research 11(2), 84–89.

Timiras, P. 2003. The nervous system: functional changes. In Timiras, P. (Ed). Physiological Basis of Aging and Geriatrics. 3rd ed. CRC Press, Boca Raton, FL.

Tortora, G. and Derrickson, B. 2007. Introduction to the Human Body: The Essentials of Anatomy and Physiology. 7th ed. John Wiley & Sons, New York, NY, pp. 301 and 302, Figures 12.11 and 12.12.

Tortora, G.J. and Derrickson, B.H. 2009. Principles of Anatomy and Physiology. 12th ed. John Wiley & Sons, New Jersey.

Waugh, A. and Grant, A. 2006. Ross and Wilson Anatomy and Physiology in Health and Illness. Churchill Livingstone Elsevier, Edinburgh.

Wolkove, N., Elkholy, O., Baltzan, M. and Palayew, M. 2007. Sleep and aging: 1. Sleep disorders commonly found in older people. Canadian Medical Association Journal 176(9), 1299–1304.

Useful websites

Parkinson's Disease Society. http://www.parkinsons.org.uk/.

Chapter 5

Breathing

Aims

After reading this chapter you will be able to discuss the normal structure and function of the systems associated with breathing.

Learning Outcomes

After completion of this chapter you will be able to:

- Describe the normal structure and function of the respiratory and cardiovascular systems
- Conduct a comprehensive patient assessment of the above systems using appropriate tools
- Detail the changes in the above systems that are associated with ageing
- Discuss the presentation and management of some common health problems related to the above systems that occur in older adults.

Introduction

We will begin this chapter with an overview of the normal anatomy and physiology of the respiratory system. After this we will examine changes within the respiratory system associated with ageing and will then consider how the health-care professional conducts an assessment of respiratory function. The common health conditions of pneumonia and influenza will be discussed and the management of these conditions will also be considered.

In addition, aspects of the cardiovascular system will also be considered in this chapter, as effective respiration is closely linked with a healthy and effective cardiovascular

---

The Physiological Effects of Ageing: Implications for Nursing Practice, First Edition
© Alistair Farley, Ella McLafferty and Charles Hendry
Published 2011 by Blackwell Publishing Ltd

system. An overview of the anatomy and physiology of the heart and circulation will be presented. Changes within the cardiovascular system associated with ageing will be reviewed and the common health condition of heart failure will be discussed and management explored.

Normal structure and function

The respiratory system consists of a number of different parts, all of which work together to enable the above functions to be carried out effectively. The respiratory system is composed of two parts: an upper and a lower respiratory tract.

Upper respiratory tract

Nose

The term 'nose' refers to the prominent feature of the face and also to the internal nasal cavity. The largest portion of the nose is composed of cartilage and bone. The bridge of the nose consists of the nasal bones plus the frontal and the maxillary bones of the skull. The nasal septum divides the cavity into two halves. The external opening is formed by the nostrils and the internal cavity is called the internal nares. The floor of the nasal cavity is formed by the hard and soft palates. The hard palate is formed by the maxillary and palatine bones of the skull, and the tissues of the soft palate extend from the hard palate. These structures allow us to eat and breathe at the same time. The soft palate rises during swallowing and blocks off the nasopharynx, thus preventing food from entering the nasal cavity. The side walls of the nasal cavity have three bony ridges, the turbinates (or conchae), which increases the surface area of mucous membrane. The mucous membrane lining of the nasal cavity is very vascular (and therefore warm). The internal nares open into the nasopharynx.

The nasal sinuses are air-filled cavities in the skull bones which open into the nose. These cavities help to reduce the weight of the skull and produce additional mucus. The mucous membrane lining the superior surface of the nose forms the olfactory epithelium which functions as the sensory organ of smell.

Pharynx

The pharynx is the common opening for both the digestive and respiratory systems; it receives air from the nose and food/fluid from the mouth. It extends from the internal nares to the larynx. It is divided into three parts, namely:

1. The nasopharynx, which contains the uvula and the Eustachian tube, and which carries air into the middle ear
2. The oro-pharynx where two sets of tonsils (lymphatic tissue) guard the fauces or entrance to the throat
3. The laryngo-pharynx which lies above the larynx and the oesophagus.

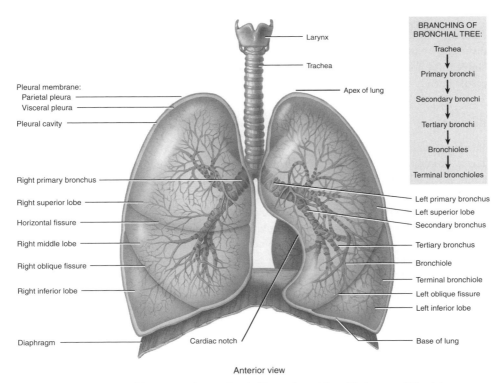

Larynx

Trachea

Apex of lung

Pleural membrane:
Parietal pleura
Visceral pleura

Pleural cavity

Right primary bronchus

Right superior lobe

Horizontal fissure

Right middle lobe

Right oblique fissure

Right inferior lobe

Diaphragm

Cardiac notch

BRANCHING OF
BRONCHIAL TREE:

Trachea
↓
Primary bronchi
↓
Secondary bronchi
↓
Tertiary bronchi
↓
Bronchioles
↓
Terminal bronchioles

Left primary bronchus
Left superior lobe
Secondary bronchus

Tertiary bronchus

Bronchiole

Terminal bronchiole
Left oblique fissure
Left inferior lobe

Base of lung

Anterior view

Figure 5.1   Diagram of lower respiratory tract. (Reproduced from Tortora and Derrickson (2007). With permission from John Wiley & Sons.)

Lower respiratory tract (Figure 5.1)

Larynx

The larynx lies below the pharynx and in front of the oesophagus. It consists of a series of cartilages connected by muscles and ligaments and lined with ciliated mucous membrane. The largest of these cartilages is the thyroid cartilage (Adam's apple). The thyroid gland lies on either side of the thyroid cartilage.

On the superior edge of the larynx is a leaf-shaped cartilage – the epiglottis which covers the larynx during swallowing and thus prevents food entering the trachea or lower airway. The lowest part of the larynx contains the vocal cords. Air from the chest causes vibration of the vocal chords. The sound created is modified by the tongue, palate and lips.

Trachea, bronchi and bronchioles

The trachea (windpipe) is $\sim$12-cm long. It extends into the chest cavity in front of the oesophagus. It consists of a series of C-shaped rings of cartilage connected by smooth muscle, and is lined by ciliated mucous membrane. The C-shaped rings maintain the lumen of the trachea, thus ensuring a patent airway. The 'open' part of the C lies posteriorly, next to the oesophagus and allows for some 'give' or movement of the oesophageal wall when we swallow.

The trachea divides at its lower end (the carina) to form the right and left bronchi which enter the lungs. The right bronchus is shorter and more vertical than the left which is slightly displaced by the heart. The bronchi divide within the lungs into smaller bronchi and bronchioles. Their structure is similar to that of the trachea, but as the bronchi divide there is less cartilage and more smooth muscle until the smallest bronchioles contain no cartilage at all.

Alveolus

The terminal bronchioles end in a cluster of air sacs called alveoli (singular – alveolus). These bronchioles and alveoli are surrounded by elastic tissue. An alveolus consists of a thin layer of squamous epithelium supported by elastic connective tissue within a thin interstitial space. These have very thin walls consisting of a single layer of cells. It is because of these thin walls that gas exchange can take place. The alveoli are surrounded by the capillaries of the pulmonary circulation. Gaseous exchange takes place between the alveoli and these blood capillaries where oxygen leaves the alveoli to enter the blood capillaries and carbon dioxide leaves these capillaries to enter the alveoli. The carbon dioxide is then exhaled. The movement of gases across the alveolar–capillary membrane takes place by diffusion. Diffusion is the movement of a dissolved substance (the solute) from an area of high concentration to an area of low concentration until there is an equal distribution. The structure and number of alveoli mean that there is a huge surface area across which diffusion takes place.

Lungs

The lungs are conical structures with the point or apex lying under each clavicle and the base resting on the diaphragm. They are divided into lobes – three in the right lung and two in the left. Each lobe is further divided into lobules which contain hundreds of alveoli (Figure 5.2). The bronchi enter the lungs at the hilum which is also the place where the blood vessels and nerves enter and leave. The lungs are supplied with blood from two sources – pulmonary arteries bringing deoxygenated blood from the right ventricle. These vessels go on to form the capillaries which surround the alveoli. It is here that oxygen is taken in and carbon dioxide given off. The other vessels, the bronchial arteries, supply oxygenated blood to the tissues of the bronchioles and lung.

The lungs are stimulated by the ANS. The parasympathetic branch is carried in the vagus nerve. Parasympathetic stimulation leads to vasoconstriction (narrowing) of the bronchioles and sympathetic stimulation leads to dilation (widening) of the bronchioles.

Pleura

This double-layered membrane surrounds the lung tissue. The inner or visceral layer is attached to the outer surface of the lungs. The outer or parietal layer is attached to the undersurface of the ribs and intercostal muscles, and the superior surface of the diaphragm. The two layers of pleura lie close together, but there is a potential space between them. This pleural space is a fluid-filled cavity which allows the pleural layers to move smoothly against one another during breathing.

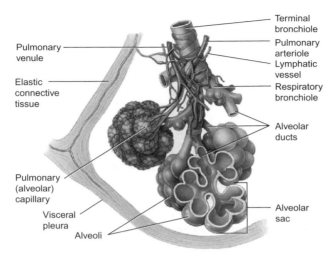

Terminal
bronchiole

Pulmonary
arteriole

Lymphatic
vessel

Respiratory
bronchiole

Alveolar
ducts

Alveolar
sac

Pulmonary
venule

Elastic
connective
tissue

Pulmonary
(alveolar)
capillary

Visceral
pleura

Alveoli

Figure 5.2 Diagram of lung lobule. (Reproduced from Nair and Peate (2009). With permission from John Wiley & Sons.)

Thoracic cavity

This is the cavity which contains most of the respiratory system. The lungs are contained within the thoracic cavity, which is bounded by the neck at the top, the diaphragm at the bottom and the sternum, ribs, spine and intercostal muscles in the circumference. The diaphragm is a sheet of involuntary muscle which separates the chest from the abdomen. It is dome shaped when relaxed and when contracted it flattens, thus increasing the size of the thoracic cavity. Two sets of intercostal muscles link one rib to the next.

Mechanics of respiration

The two sets of intercostal muscles are the external and internal intercostals. The external intercostals, when contracted, pull the ribs outward and upward. This enlarges the circumference of the thoracic cavity, that is, from front to back. Relaxation of these muscles allows the thoracic cavity to return to its original shape and size. The internal intercostals are only used during forced expiration such as strenuous activity or blowing up a balloon. Contraction of these muscles squeezes more air out of the lungs than is needed during normal respiration, giving a forced expiration.

The mechanics of breathing

Inspiration

For inspiration to occur, the pressure within the lungs must fall below atmospheric pressure. This occurs as a result of the contraction of the diaphragm and external intercostal muscles. This contraction increases the size of the thorax causing the lungs to expand (contraction of the diaphragm increases the size of the thorax from top to bottom, whilst contraction of the external intercostals increases the size of the thorax from back to front). When the lungs expand, the pressure within them decreases (intrapulmonic pressure) due to Boyle's law, and a pressure gradient is formed. Boyle's law states that pressure is inversely proportional to volume, that is, as the volume increases within the thoracic cavity, the pressure decreases. Atmospheric pressure is now greater than intrapulmonic pressure, and air rushes into the lungs until intrapulmonic pressure equals that of atmospheric pressure. The process of inspiration is an active one, that is, it requires energy, or to put it another way, breathing is work.

During quiet breathing, the diaphragm and external intercostals relax, decreasing the size of the thorax. The ribcage moves downwards and inwards, and as the diaphragm moves upwards, the size of the thoracic cavity is decreased. The tension is taken off the pleura and the elastic tissue of the lungs recoils. The pressure within the lungs (intrapulmonic pressure) increases and a pressure gradient is formed. Intrapulmonic pressure becomes greater than atmospheric pressure. Air now flows out from the lungs until these two pressures are equal.

Oxygen in the lungs is not yet available to the tissues. External respiration is the process by which gases are exchanged between the alveoli and the blood in the pulmonary capillaries. The process is brought about by the difference in pressures between gases in the alveoli and in the pulmonary capillaries. Atmospheric air is composed of three main gases: nitrogen (N), oxygen (O) and carbon dioxide (CO_2). Nitrogen is an inert gas and only the levels of oxygen and carbon dioxide are important in respiration.

Not all the air we breathe in reaches the alveoli. The air passages (nose, pharynx, larynx, trachea, bronchi and bronchioles) contain air which does not reach the alveoli. These parts of the respiratory system which do not take part in gas exchange are referred to as dead space. In adults, the size of this dead space is $\sim$150 ml (Waugh and Grant, 2006).

Expiration

During forceful expiration, the rate and depth of respirations are increased as the expiratory centre is activated. Impulses are now sent to the expiratory muscles – internal intercostals and the abdominal muscles. Both these groups now contract and expiration is more forced than when passive recoil occurs alone. The lungs are prevented from recoiling too far because of the pleura. Since the layers of the pleura remain in contact with one another and the parietal layer is attached to the thoracic wall, the lungs will be limited in the extent to which they can recoil.

During normal quiet breathing, $\sim$400–500 ml of air is inspired and expired. This is called the tidal volume. However, there are times when this amount is insufficient, such as when exercising or when someone has a respiratory disease.

The inspiratory reserve volume is the extra amount of air you can breathe in over and above the tidal volume, that is, after taking a normal breath, continue to breathe in for as long as you can. Men average about 3.3 l as their inspiratory reserve volume and women average about 1.9 l.

The expiratory reserve volume is the extra amount of air you can breathe out over and above the tidal volume, that is, at the end of a breath, breathe out as far as you can. Men average about 1.0 l as their expiratory reserve volume and women average about 0.7 l.

The reason that the figures for inspiratory reserve volume is not the same as for expiratory reserve volume is that the lungs never completely empty. Even after breathing out forcefully, the lungs still contain about 1 l of air. This is called the residual volume.

The inspiratory capacity is the maximum amount of air you can breathe in = tidal volume + inspiratory reserve volume.

The vital capacity is the maximum amount of air you can breathe out after the lungs have been filled to their maximum extent = inspiratory reserve volume + tidal volume + expiratory reserve volume.

The total lung capacity is the vital capacity + residual volume. In men this averages out as 6 l and in women it is 4.2 l.

Gas exchange

As stated earlier, the walls of both alveoli and pulmonary capillaries are very closely associated with one another making diffusion easier. Diseases such as pneumonia cause the alveolar–pulmonary membrane to thicken, making gas exchange more difficult. The structure and number of alveoli mean that there is a huge surface area across which diffusion has to take place.

Oxygen and carbon dioxide transport

Blood returning to the lungs from the right ventricle is deoxygenated blood, that is, it has given up some of its oxygen to the tissues. The pO_2 in this blood is lower than the pO_2 in the alveoli. (Remember, gas at a higher concentration/pressure will move by diffusion to an area of lower concentration/pressure.) Therefore, oxygen moves from the alveoli into the blood.

In contrast, carbon dioxide levels in the blood returning to the lungs are higher than those within the alveoli, and therefore carbon dioxide diffuses from the blood out into the alveoli. It is then expired on the exhaled breath.

Control of breathing

Breathing for the most part is an involuntary action; however, this can be overridden by voluntary control if and when necessary, for example, breathing is under voluntary control when we speak and form words and sentences. The main control of respiration is the result of the interplay of a number of different elements. These include:

- Nervous system control
- Chemical control
- Other factors.

Nervous system control

As with many vital functions, the control of breathing is located in the brainstem, namely the medulla oblongata and the pons varolii.

Within the medulla can be found the respiratory centre which is also known as the medullary rhythmicity centre. This sets the basic pattern of breathing. The respiratory centre can be subdivided into inspiratory and expiratory areas.

The inspiratory centre (primary respiratory pacemaker) exhibits an intrinsic excitability that sends nerve impulses along the phrenic and intercostal nerves. These cause the diaphragm and the external intercostal muscles to contract, thus increasing the thoracic volume. At the same time, the inspiratory centre sends an inhibitory impulse to the expiratory centre, thus ensuring that only inspiration can occur. It is important to note that inspiration is always an active process that requires energy.

The expiratory centre is normally inactive during quiet respiration, and expiration is therefore a passive process dependent upon the elastic recoil of the diaphragm and external intercostal muscles. However, it becomes active when there is a need to increase the rate and/or depth of respiration. When active, impulses travel along the intercostal nerve to the internal intercostal muscles and also to the abdominal muscles. When the internal intercostal muscles contract, the ribcage is pulled downwards and inwards. When the abdominal muscles contract, intra-abdominal pressure increases causing the diaphragm to move upwards. Both of these actions increase the intra-thoracic pressure forcing air out of the lungs. During expiration, inspiration is inhibited. Normal quiet breathing consists of repeated cycles of inspiration, expiration and short pause. Inspiration lasts ~2 seconds and expiration 3 seconds (Seeley et al., 2003; Waugh and Grant, 2006).

Chemical control

In addition to the nervous control of breathing, the body also responds to a number of changes in body chemistry.

Chemoreceptors are specialised nerve cells which respond to chemicals that become attached to receptors on their cell membranes. In respiration, these include chemoreceptors in the carotid artery and aorta, and a chemosensitive area in the medulla. The chemoreceptors found in the carotid artery and the aorta are sensitive to changes in blood CO_2 and O_2 levels as well as hydrogen ion concentration (H^+). However, it should be noted that these chemoreceptors are only sensitive to large decreases in O_2 level of ~50%. At this level, hypoxia will then have a large stimulatory effect on respiration.

The medullary chemosensitive area is activated by changes in CO_2 and H^+, with oxygen having no direct effect on this area. Excess CO_2 and H^+ stimulate both inspiratory and expiratory centres, thereby increasing the rate and depth of respiration.

Due to the very soluble nature of CO_2, the medullary area is able to detect very small changes in this respiratory gas, and thus it is CO_2 concentration and not O_2 that is the key influence over normal breathing.

It may be useful to consider the following equation:

$$CO_2 + H_2O \leftrightarrow H_2CO_3 \leftrightarrow H^+ + HCO_3^-$$

In the body, carbon dioxide will combine with water to produce carbonic acid. This can then break down to produce hydrogen ions and bicarbonate ions.

It can be seen from the above equation that a rise in pCO_2 will result in an increase in H^+, thus lowering pH. If pCO_2 rises above normal, then the body can compensate by increasing the respiratory rate and depth, thereby increasing the excretion of CO_2. This moves the above equation to the left, thus 'locking' some of the H^+ up in carbonic acid and therefore maintaining blood pH within normal limits.

This reaction is reversible as seen by the double-headed arrows and can occur as:

$$H^+ + HCO_3^- \leftrightarrow H_2CO_3 \leftrightarrow H_2O + CO_2$$

The reaction is facilitated by the enzyme carbonic anhydrase.

It should be noted that the renal system also has a role to play in maintaining a normal pH. It does this by secretion and selective re-absorption of $H^+ + HCO_3^-$.

Ageing changes in the respiratory system

The respiratory system starts to decline well before the age of 60. A gradual decline is observed in the respiratory system from the age of about 25 years, having reached its functional peak by around the age of 20 years (De Martinis and Timiras, 2003). There are a number of variables that influence the extent and speed of age-related changes in structure and function, which include intrinsic factors such as the presence of disease and extrinsic factors that include nutrition, physical exercise and smoking (De Martinis and Timiras, 2003). However, changes due to ageing are relatively insignificant when compared to the continuous effects of the external environment. If optimal growth in lung function is attained, there should be sufficient spare capacity for a decrease in lung function to have little effect as long as an older adult remains free from disease (Dyer and Stockley, 2006). The majority of older adults are therefore able to sustain their lifestyle and a satisfactory level of respiratory function that meets their needs under resting conditions (De Martinis and Timiras, 2003).

Changes in the structure of the respiratory tract

The respiratory tract is affected by ageing changes associated with the musculoskeletal system. Musculoskeletal changes account for alterations in the size and shape of the nose where the nose becomes longer and its tip begins to sag. This sagging is due to a weakening of the support offered by the upper and lower cartilages. These physical changes can impede the airflow through the nasal passages, as a result of which older adults may experience symptoms of blockage in their nose.

In addition to these musculoskeletal changes, the number of sub-mucosal glands decreases. The upper respiratory tract normally produces a nasal mucus which is thick and tenacious (Sheahan and Musialowski, 2001). This mucus is produced by goblet cells within the respiratory tract. Other glands, called sub-mucosal serous glands, produce a thin and watery mucus. In adulthood, there is a balance between the amount of thick tenacious mucus and thin watery mucus that is produced. However, with ageing, this balance is lost and a larger amount of thick, tenacious mucus is produced while there is a decrease in watery thin mucus production. This results in mucus becoming even thicker and more likely to lodge in the nasopharynx. Older adults may therefore experience recurrent coughs as they try to clear the nasopharynx. Accompanying these changes is a decrease in blood flow to the nasal area which further dries secretions which can crust leading to a sense of nasal stuffiness (Sheahan and Musialowski, 2001).

In addition to the imbalance between the production of thick, tenacious mucus and thin watery mucus, the ageing process also affects muco-ciliary clearance, where the cilia lining the trachea and the smaller airways flatten, making it much more difficult to clear secretions from the lungs. There is also a decreased ability to cough up secretions as we age (Roach, 2001). In addition to having fewer mucous-producing cells, there is a decline in the normal bronchial secretion production which may cause epithelial damage and the risk of bacteria sticking to the bronchial walls (Dyer and Stockley, 2006).

The thoracic cage and muscular function

The costal cartilages, which connect the ribs to the sternum, the ribs to each other and also to the thoracic vertebrae become more rigid and stiff resulting in decreased compliance during quiet respiration (Roach, 2001). This change increases the need to use the accessory muscles for breathing. However, the strength in the respiratory muscles begins to decrease from about the age of 55 (Sheahan and Musialowski, 2001). The intercostal muscles that help move the chest wall atrophy and become weaker, so that the work of breathing is increased. As the intercostal muscles weaken and the ribcage becomes stiffer, the diaphragm plays a larger role in breathing, as it takes over a higher proportion of the mechanical effort needed for increasing ventilation (De Martinis and Timiras, 2003).

Dyspnoea on exertion is common among older people. Whether this is due to a decrease in muscle strength or an increase in thoracic stiffness and loss of lung compliance is unclear. However, it is evident that older adults' respirations are shallower with increased diaphragmatic motion because of ageing changes in the costal structures, as described earlier when compared with younger adults (De Martinis and Timiras, 2003).

A number of changes occur with ageing in respiratory muscles (De Martinis and Timiras, 2003), namely:

- Muscle strength is decreased
- More prone to fatigue when the work of breathing is increased
- Atrophy of some respiratory muscles
- Ratio of anaerobic to aerobic metabolism is increased
- Blood supply to muscle is decreased.

Alveoli

With ageing, the structure of the alveoli also changes. The alveolar surface of a younger adult is $\sim 70 \, m^2$ (Tortora and Derrickson, 2009). Sheahan and Musialowski (2001) suggest that this large surface area for gas exchange reduces with age. The alveoli themselves become shallower and flatten as a result of the loss of septal tissue (De Martinis and Timiras, 2003). The walls of the alveoli become thinner, and there is a decrease in the number of capillaries surrounding each alveolus. The alveolar ducts become stretched, resulting in the alveoli enlarging or tearing. However, the number of alveoli remains relatively constant. The changes in the structure of the alveoli can be attributed to changes in the elastic fibre network of the alveolar walls. There is also some evidence that the alveolar changes including the increased alveolar duct size, the reduction in surface area and decreased diffusing capacity could be related to the disruption of collagen fibres within them (Dyer and Stockley, 2006).

The pattern of air distribution alters with age, resulting in an increase in alveolar duct air but a decrease in alveolar air. From the age of 30, there is a decrease in alveolar air of 4% for each subsequent decade. As oxygen transport is most efficient in the alveoli, the decrease in alveolar air space will result in reducing optimal oxygen diffusion from alveolar air into pulmonary capillaries (De Martinis and Timiras, 2003). The reduction in oxygen movement from alveolus to pulmonary capillary may reduce overall oxygen concentration within the blood, thereby making the older adult more prone to hypoxia after little effort.

Elastic recoil

The lungs begin to distend as the elastic tissue stretches and elastic recoil decreases. Normal expiration is mostly a passive process that is attributable to recoil of the elastic tissue of the stretched lungs and thorax. However, the amount of elastic tissue decreases with the ageing process while the amount of fibrous tissue is increased. Not only does the amount of elastic tissue decrease, but also the alteration in its distribution has an effect on lung function, in that abnormal location or structure of the elastic fibres may contribute to impairment of ventilation and perfusion of the lungs. Collagen becomes more rigid and changes in its structure together with changes in elastin contribute to the loss of recoil.

Control of ventilation

The action of the carotid body and aortic body chemoreceptors appear to be less responsive to changes in blood oxygen and pH levels with advancing age (Roach, 2001). The respiratory centres in the brain located within the pons and the medulla may also be significantly less efficient in older people (De Martinis and Timiras, 2003). The ventilatory response to hypoxia is decreased by 51% in healthy men between the ages of 64 and 73 compared with healthy men between the ages of 22 and 30 (Roach, 2001). Older people are therefore less able to tolerate hypoxia or hypercapnia (Sheahan and Musialowski, 2001).

Changes in ventilation with ageing

Pulmonary ventilatory function steadily decreases after the age of 50. Changes in compliance within the respiratory system result in premature airway closure and poorly ventilated or unventilated alveoli at resting lung volumes. Small airways are more likely to collapse in the lung bases because of reduced elastic recoil. As a result of decreased elastic lung recoil, the bases of the lungs do not inflate well and secretions that collect in the lungs are not so easily expectorated.

Vital capacity, maximum ventilation rate and gas exchange all decrease with age. However, these effects are largely negated due to large reserve capacity in the respiratory system. Vital capacity decreases as the ability to fill and empty the lungs is reduced (weakening of respiratory muscles and stiffness of cartilage and ribs). As a result, maximum minute ventilation rates are reduced; this limits the person's capacity for intense exercise. The decreased vital capacity of the lung that occurs with ageing is also thought to be associated with height and posture changes. While vital capacity decreases, the residual volume increases.

An increase in the diameter of the bronchioles and alveolar ducts leads to an increase in dead space which reduces the amount of air available for gas exchange. Partial alveolar wall collapse and thickening of the alveolar membrane further reduces gas exchange across the respiratory surface. However, oxygen requirements are generally less because of lower basal metabolism in older people (Dyer and Stockley, 2006). Blood gas levels of pO_2 may fall slightly with ageing, but arterial pCO_2 levels stay approximately the same.

With ageing, the respiratory system cannot accommodate the increased metabolic rate during exercise. Consequently, there is a greater increase in ventilation for a similar increase in workload compared to younger adults (Sheahan and Musialowski, 2001).

Exercise can delay the ageing changes associated with the mechanical properties of the lungs. Physical training can increase respiratory muscle function, maximal voluntary ventilation, maximal minute ventilation and static lung volumes. Ageing appears to affect lung tissue mechanics to a lesser degree than it does to chest wall dynamics. There is no evidence to suggest that habitual physical activity counteracts age-related changes in chest wall mechanics.

Assessing respiratory function

The nurse must be able to carry out a comprehensive respiratory assessment. Upon approaching the patient, the nurse should assess the rhythm, rate and depth of breathing. The patient's colour should be noted, although on its own this is not a very reliable indicator of a patient's respiratory status. Simple observation can also indicate use of accessory muscles of breathing or evidence of breathlessness (dyspnoea). The neck and back should be assessed for structural defects, such as deviation of the trachea, kyphosis or scoliosis – all of which interfere with, and limit, chest expansion.

The nurse should enquire whether the patient has had to limit their levels of activity or has been limited in their exercise tolerance due to breathing difficulties. The degree of breathlessness can be established by identifying the level of breathlessness:

1. Shortness of breath when hurrying on a level surface or when walking up hills or stairs
2. Shortness of breath when walking on a level surface with people of the same age
3. Shortness of breath when walking on a level surface at one's own pace
4. Shortness of breath when washing or dressing
5. Shortness of breath when sitting quietly.

(Taken from Heath and Schofield, 1999, p. 126)

Another indicator of the extent of breathlessness is the distance the older person can walk on a flat surface without stopping to rest. Patients should also be asked if they have shortness of breath during the night or at specific times and also asked if breathlessness interferes with their lifestyle.

A smoking history should be taken including any attempts or desire to stop smoking. This should include a past and present history of smoking. The age that the person started smoking and the number of cigarettes smoked daily should be noted.

Any history of coughing should be identified, taking particular note of the time of day, and whether productive or not. Amount, if any, and type of phlegm should be noted. Also identify how long the cough has been present and the colour of the phlegm if present.

Exposure to pollutants should be acknowledged, and if people live in an industrial area where there are high emissions of environmental pollutants, this should be noted. Present and past occupations and hobbies may also indicate contact with possible respiratory irritants. Staff should also enquire if other factors such as cold, damp conditions or air conditioning aggravate the problem.

Common respiratory problems associated with ageing

In this section, we will examine a number of common conditions of the respiratory tract particularly associated with ageing.

Pneumonia

Pneumonia is a serious and life-threatening condition in older people. The death rate associated with pneumonia is estimated to be five times higher in older people over 65 when compared to people under the age of 65. In older populations, the condition usually requires a period of hospitalisation. Coexisting long-term illnesses may complicate the situation.

Pneumonia can be caused by a variety of factors including bacteria, viruses, fungi and aspiration of fluids (Mauk, 2006). It is an inflammation of the lungs usually caused by infection and is often associated with the alveoli filling with fluid, that is, to consolidate. This accumulation of exudate within the alveoli compromises gas exchange and can result in death. If the pneumonia has a patchy distribution, it is referred to as bronchopneumonia. Lobar pneumonia refers to a single segment or an entire lobe of lung affected. Older adults are particularly susceptible to this condition due to their reduced immune response associated with ageing changes, the possible existence of pre-existing respiratory illness, a reduced cough reflex and a reduction in levels of mobility (Meiner and Lueckenotte, 2006). The most common type affecting older adults is bacterial pneumonia (Roach, 2001).

Typical symptoms of bacterial pneumonia include cough, fever, sweating, shivering, loss of appetite and a feeling of being unwell. Headaches, and general aches and pains are also common. Sputum production increases and this may become yellow/green in colour. Occasionally, the sputum is bloodstained. The patient can become breathless, tachypnoeic and develop chest tightness. Pleuritic pain may develop which is often worse on inspiration.

However, pneumonia may manifest itself differently in older people when compared to younger people. Older people may exhibit increased respiratory rate and increased pulse rate as the first symptom with respirations consistently over 26–28 per minute. Additional symptoms include a general deterioration and changes in mental status. Typical symptoms of cough, chest pain, production of sputum and fever are not always present, making pneumonia difficult to detect in older patients (Roach, 2001). Older adults may also demonstrate symptoms of dehydration and confusion (Meiner and Lueckenotte, 2006).

Viral pneumonia symptoms are initially similar to influenza symptoms, with fever, a dry cough, headache, muscular pain and a generalised weakness. Within 24 hours, there is increasing breathlessness, a worsening cough and a small amount of mucus may be produced. Pyrexia is common. Viral pneumonias may be complicated by secondary bacterial invasion, leading to a picture similar to that seen in bacterial pneumonia.

Diagnosis is confirmed with chest X-ray, sputum culture and full blood count. Clinical history and examination should always be obtained. Auscultation may demonstrate 'crackles' in the lungs.

Viral pneumonia generally clears by itself, but bacterial pneumonia will require appropriate antibiotic therapy. The causative agent should be identified by obtaining a sputum sample and sending it for culture and sensitivity to determine the antibiotic of choice. The duration of therapy is also dictated by the nature of infection and responses to treatment; however, antibiotic therapy is generally administered for 10–14 days as required (Meiner and Lueckenotte, 2006). Adequate levels of hydration (1500–2000 ml/day) should be maintained, nutritional status assessed and adequate nutrition given. Sufficient rest is also helpful. Complications following respiratory illness often lead to death in older people (Mauk, 2006). Older adults should therefore be reminded to contact their health-care professional if their respiratory status does not improve.

The older adult should consider the annual influenza vaccination as pneumonia is often a complication of influenza. A one-off vaccine against pneumonia is also available for them.

Management of the older adult with pneumonia

Vital signs (temperature, pulse, blood pressure and respirations) should be monitored as frequently as the patient's condition dictates. Any increase in respiratory and/or pulse rate should be reported to senior staff. Staff should also examine the patient's nail beds, lips and oral mucosa for evidence of cyanosis and record their findings. Sputum should be monitored for amount, colour, consistency and presence of blood.

Regular pain assessment is required to identify and treat any pleuritic pain or pain associated with coughing. Analgesia should be administered as prescribed and evaluated for effectiveness.

Patients should also be assessed for restlessness, confusion and drowsiness as they may be an indication of decreased oxygenation of the brain. Oxygen saturation should be monitored closely. A reduction of oxygenated blood flow to the brain is closely linked to delirium.

Patients with pneumonia may report fatigue, decreased activity tolerance and loss of appetite. Activities should therefore be planned to alternate with rest periods in order to prevent exhaustion. Assistance with activities such as personal hygiene needs and personal care will also reduce the risk of fatigue. Meals offered should be nutritious, small and frequent with assistance being offered as required. A quiet environment will do much to promote rest and sleep.

It may be necessary to administer supplemental oxygen to an older adult with pneumonia in order to correct dyspnoea and hypoxia. Oxygen is a gas that is present in air at a concentration of 21%. Pharmacologically, oxygen is a prescription only medication under the Medicines Act 1968, and therefore, except in an emergency, oxygen should always be prescribed by a medical practitioner.

Oxygen can be delivered in a variety of ways. The most usual means of administering oxygen are by facemask or nasal cannulae. Nasal cannulae have the advantage of allowing the person to eat, drink and speak without interrupting the delivery of oxygen (Jevon and Ewens, 2001).

When administering oxygen, safety issues are of paramount concern. The nurse should promote and ensure patient safety during the administration of oxygen and adhere to local policies, guidelines and national protocols as appropriate (Francis, 2006). Oxygen will support combustion and therefore must not be used near a naked flame or sources of static electricity. White soft paraffin or other oil-based products or face creams should not be used to relieve dryness or soreness to the nose as these products are potentially combustible. Furthermore, these have a tendency to clog nasal cannulae. It is important to reassess the patient frequently to confirm that they continue to receive the prescribed dose of oxygen and that the mask or cannulae remain in position and comfortable (Jevon and Ewens, 2001).

To avoid the drying effects of oxygen, humidification should be used whenever possible and the nurse should ensure a good fit of the mask or nasal cannulae. The patient should be encouraged to drink between 1500 and 2000 ml of fluids to maintain good hydration and to help loosen bronchial secretions (Roach, 2001). Oral hygiene should be offered to the patient receiving oxygen as they may experience drying of the mouth.

It is important that the nurse establishes a good rapport with the patient in order to offer support and reassurance regarding their oxygen therapy. Additionally, the nurse should ensure that the patient has a good understanding of the reasons for the prescription of oxygen. Where appropriate, this should also include relatives and carers (Jevon and Ewens, 2001). This will help maintain patient compliance with this potentially demanding therapy.

 Point for Practice

Hamish, aged 78, is due to be discharged home and to continue oxygen therapy at home. Outline a plan of care to prepare Hamish and his family for this therapy.

Correct patient positioning can help to maximise air entry and gas exchange. When sitting upright, gravity pulls the abdominal contents down towards the pelvis and away from the diaphragm thus allowing freer movement of the diaphragm. When lying down (and especially in obese people), the abdominal contents compress or splint the diaphragm thus reducing lung expansion. Correct positioning will also allow freer movement of the ribcage. Breathless patients, therefore, benefit from sitting in an upright or semi-recumbent position. This may also be necessary when sleeping. Frequent position changes will aid in the prevention of pressure sore development whilst assisting with lung expansion and removal of bronchial secretions.

The physiotherapist is a key health-care professional in the management of breathlessness. They can assist the patient to improve gas exchange through a breathlessness management 'package of care'. Auscultation of the chest may reveal decreased breath sounds, over the affected areas, wheezing, crackles or gurgles. Physiotherapy can also assist the patient to cough effectively and expectorate sputum. Chest physiotherapy percussion and postural drainage can also be performed if required. Splinting painful areas with a pillow may decrease discomfort while coughing. Naso-tracheal suctioning may be required if the patient is unable to clear their airway by coughing. Nurses and other health-care professionals need to be familiar with the instructions and techniques used by the physiotherapist in order to support the patient. One of the supportive measures that nurses can encourage patients to engage in is to breathe deeply every 1–2 hours to facilitate maximum expansion of the lungs (Roach, 2001).

 Point for Practice

What interventions could you use to assist a client/patient to expectorate sputum?

Influenza

Influenza viruses cause respiratory illness. This condition is most prevalent in the United Kingdom during the winter months. It is highly contagious, easily transmissible and dangerous for older people (Roach, 2001). For most adults the illness runs its course, however, for older people the condition can be much more severe and can lead to death .The typical incubation period is 2–3 days and people can remain infectious for another 3–5 days (While et al., 2005). The virus is quickly spread by droplet infection. The influenza virus attaches to a host cell, penetrates the cell membrane and replicates inside the cell. Over a 6-hour period, one infected virus particle can create 1 million identical virus particles (While et al., 2005). These virus particles quickly destroy cells in the respiratory tract. This rapidity of destruction leads to the suddenness in the onset of flu symptoms.

During flu epidemics, the vast majority of those who die (up to 90%) are over the age of 65 (Banning, 2005; Lueckenotte, 2000). Vaccination programmes have been highly effective in reducing the numbers of those succumbing to the infection and the uptake of these vaccinations is gradually increasing (Balicer et al., 2005; While et al., 2005). There are different strains of influenza and the prediction of the strain most likely to lead to an outbreak of influenza dictates which vaccine will be made available. Barriers to the effectiveness of the vaccine include poor match between the vaccine and circulating strains and poor antibody response of older patients. All adults over 65 should have the yearly flu vaccine before the onset of winter (Roach, 2001) as it takes 1–2 weeks to develop antibody protection after receiving the flu vaccine (Lueckenotte, 2000).

However, a small number of older people refuse to participate in vaccination programmes. Reasons for non-participation are varied and include older people's beliefs about their own health and their perceptions of being low risk of developing influenza. Many actually believe that the vaccine contributes to them developing influenza and some are simply not interested in being vaccinated (Mangtani et al., 2006). Some older people also refuse vaccination because they feel it is ageist and discriminatory to vaccinate people simply on the grounds of their age (Evans et al., 2007).

However, many older people will accept the vaccination if it is recommended by a health-care worker (Mangtani et al., 2006). Therefore in view of informed consent it is the nurse's role, when working with older people, to explore their beliefs about influenza, their risks of developing it and the perceived benefits of participating in the yearly vaccination programme. Side effects to the vaccination are possible including development of viral pneumonia but this is a rare complication.

Symptoms of influenza include an abrupt onset of fever, chills, shivering, headache, generalised aching of the back, arms and legs, fatigue, cough, sore throat, nasal congestion and loss of appetite (Banning, 2005; Lueckenotte, 2000). Signs and symptoms may last up to 14 days from the onset of the infection. Body temperature can increase to 40°C for 2–3 days. Chills, fever and aching joints are less common in older people (Roach, 2001). However, sputum production and dyspnoea are more common (Banning, 2005) and older people are at risk of developing pneumonia as a secondary infection.

It may be difficult to recognise influenza in older adults. The typical signs associated with this condition may be subdued or absent. Changes in mental status, exacerbation of any underlying conditions and a below normal temperature may indicate infection in older people. Subnormal temperature accompanied by hypotension; rapid pulse; cool and clammy skin are signs of sepsis in older people (Lueckenotte, 2000).

Management of influenza includes assessment of hydration and ensuring that the patient drinks at least 1500–2000 ml of fluid daily to combat dehydration related to pyrexia. Oral aspirin or paracetamol may be administered to relieve discomfort and help reduce pyrexia (Lueckenotte, 2000). Non-steroidal anti-inflammatory drugs may be given for muscular aches and pains. Rest in bed is very important to combat the feelings of fatigue and weakness. If the individual is in hospital, then vital signs should be monitored and recorded. Meals that are easily digestible and nutritious should be provided. Antibiotics may be necessary if there are any signs and symptoms of secondary bacterial infection (Roach, 2001). There are two antiviral drugs recommended by NICE (2003), which are effective in the treatment of influenza but they must be administered within 48 hours after the onset of symptoms of influenza to be of any benefit in shortening and reducing the severity of the illness (Banning, 2005; Roach, 2001).

There are a number of complications associated with influenza including development of bronchitis, otitis media, sinusitis, viral pneumonia, neurological or arthritic conditions. The symptoms of viral pneumonia will commence within 24 hours of fever. The patient will develop a dry cough which later produces bloodstained sputum, tachypnoea will be evident, diffuse crackles in the lungs can be heard, progressive cyanosis can be observed and respiratory failure can develop (Banning, 2005). Not every patient will develop complications of influenza, but the role of the nurse is also to monitor and record any signs of complications and report these to senior staff.

Cardiovascular system

 Revision Point

Using a resource of your choice, revise:

- The structure of blood vessels
- The pulmonary and systemic circulations.

Normal structure and function

The heart is located between the two lungs in the mediastinum of the thoracic cavity. It is more or less in the centre of the thorax being slanted diagonally with approximately two-thirds of its mass to the left of the body's midline. The heart lies closer to the front of the thorax than to the back. A person's heart is about the same size as their closed fist.

The heart is described as being cone-shaped with the pointed end known as the apex which is normally situated about the level of the fifth intercostal space, or the space between the fifth and sixth ribs. The uppermost part is known as the base and is formed mostly by the left atrium. Major blood vessels of the heart enter and leave at the base. The base is in a relatively fixed position because of the attachments to these great vessels but the apex is able to move.

The heart is surrounded and protected by a membrane known as the pericardium which consists of two layers – the fibrous pericardium and the serous pericardium. The fibrous layer fixes the heart within the mediastinum. The serous layer is divided into a visceral and parietal layer. The visceral layer (sometimes known as the epicardium) adheres tightly to the surface of the heart (Tortora and Grabowski, 2004). Between these two layers is a small amount of serous fluid known as pericardial fluid. This prevents friction between these layers when the heart is beating.

The heart wall is composed of three layers. The epicardium is the thin, transparent outer layer of the heart wall. The epicardium and the visceral layer of the pericardium are two names for the same structure (Seeley et al., 2003).

The myocardium is the middle layer of the heart wall and is composed of cardiac muscle tissue. Cardiac muscle is special. It is under involuntary control and the muscle fibres are arranged in such a way that it is unnecessary to stimulate each one separately in order for contraction of the muscle fibres to take place. The myocardium acts as a coordinated unit which allows action potentials to be transmitted from one cell to another. This allows all the cells in the atria to contract in unison followed by a similar pattern in the ventricles. Contraction of the myocardium creates the force necessary to pump blood around the lungs and the body. Cardiac muscle has an intrinsic ability to contract without receiving any external stimuli. This is located in a collection of tissue known as the conduction system.

The endocardium is a thin layer of endothelial tissue. This is a connective tissue lining the inside of the heart and is continuous with the blood vessels that enter and leave the heart. It is very smooth, and this property helps to reduce the chance of a blood clot (thrombosis) forming within the heart or blood vessels.

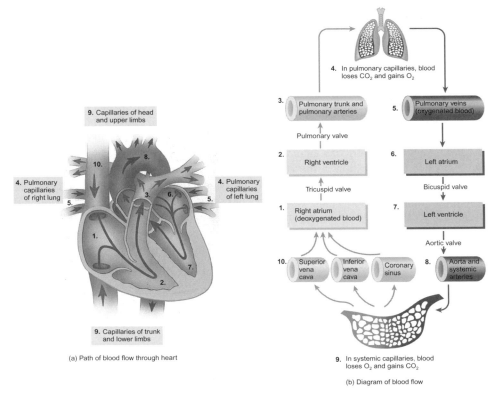

9. Capillaries of head and upper limbs

10.

8.

4. Pulmonary capillaries of right lung

5.

4. Pulmonary capillaries of left lung

5.

1.

3. 6.

7.

2.

9. Capillaries of trunk and lower limbs

(a) Path of blood flow through heart

4. In pulmonary capillaries, blood loses CO_2 and gains O_2

3. Pulmonary trunk and pulmonary arteries

5. Pulmonary veins (oxygenated blood)

Pulmonary valve

2. Right ventricle

6. Left atrium

Tricuspid valve

Bicuspid valve

1. Right atrium (deoxygenated blood)

7. Left ventricle

Aortic valve

10. Superior vena cava | Inferior vena cava | Coronary sinus

8. Aorta and systemic arteries

9. In systemic capillaries, blood loses O_2 and gains CO_2

(b) Diagram of blood flow

Figure 5.3   Diagram of blood flow through the heart. (Reproduced from Tortora and Derrickson (2007). With permission from John Wiley & Sons.)

Blood flow (Figure 5.3)

The heart is in effect two pumps. The right heart pumps blood through the pulmonary circulation: deoxygenated blood enters the right atrium via the superior and inferior venae cavae. It passes through the tricuspid valve entering the right ventricle before being ejected through the pulmonary valve into the pulmonary artery. The blood circulates through the lungs where it loses carbon dioxide and gains oxygen. Oxygenated blood now enters the left side of the heart. The left heart pumps blood through the systemic circulation. Blood enters the left atrium via the pulmonary veins. The blood passes through the bicuspid (mitral) valve into the left ventricle. When the heart contracts the blood is ejected through the aortic valve into the aorta.

 Revision Point

Many older people have problems maintaining a normal blood pressure, for example, postural hypotension and hypertension. Revise the mechanisms by which a normal blood pressure is maintained and how this may change with ageing.

Changes in the cardiovascular system of the older adult

Heart failure

Heart failure is a disorder in which the heart loses its ability to pump blood efficiently throughout the body. It has been defined as a 'Complex syndrome that can result from any structural or functional cardiac disorder that impairs the ability of the heart to respond to physiological demands for increased cardiac output' (SIGN 95, 2007, p. 1).

Heart failure may affect the left, right or both sides of the heart. If the left side of the heart fails (left ventricular failure), then fluid (pulmonary oedema) will build up in the lungs due to congestion of the veins of the lungs. If the right side of the heart fails (right ventricular failure), general body vein pressure will increase and fluid (generalised oedema) will accumulate in the body, especially the tissues of the legs and abdominal organs (of these, the liver is the organ most likely to be affected).

Heart failure can be caused by a number of different diseases and conditions, and can occur either as an acute event or as a chronic, long-standing condition. SIGN (2007) state that these causes include:

- Ischaemic heart disease
- Hypertension
- Diseases of the heart valves
- Cardiomyopathy.

Heart failure is a chronic illness occurring mostly in older men (NICE, CG5, 2003), characterised by an unpredictable path causing distressing clinical signs and symptoms, recurrent hospitalisations and a higher mortality than some cancers (e.g. breast and prostate cancer) (Quinn et al., 2001).

Heart failure is expected to double with each decade of life after the age of 45 (Davis et al., 2000) and in the future will be more prominent in those greater than 70 years of age (Jaarsma et al., 2006; NICE, CG5, 2003).

In the United Kingdom, ~900 000 people have been diagnosed with heart failure (Petersen et al., 2002) and it is expected that with the growth in the population of older people over the next 20 years, the extent of this disabling disease will worsen.

Heart failure has high morbidity and mortality rates (Watson, 2009). One month after the initial diagnosis, heart failure is associated with a 15% mortality rate (Cowie et al., 2002) and 3 months following an index hospital admission 20% of patients have been readmitted with heart failure and 13% have died (Cleland et al., 2003). At 6 months, following a new diagnosis of heart failure, it has been reported that between 18% and 47% of newly diagnosed heart failure patients are readmitted to hospital with worsening heart failure (Cowie et al., 2002; Davis et al., 2000). Heart failure tends to present itself in the 70 years plus age group, the majority of whom have other co-morbidities to deal with such as high blood pressure, diabetes, COPD and renal impairment (De Geest et al., 2004).

Other influential factors such as sensory and cognitive impairment have also been identified as being prevalent in older patients with heart failure which can impact significantly on adherence to specific medication regimes and can result in additional demands on these partners/family members (De Geest et al., 2003).

Clinical features

Left-sided heart failure:

- Shortness of breath together with a reduction in mobility.
- In less severe cases, breathing problems only occur upon exertion.
- A chronic dry cough may develop.
- Fatigue.

Right-sided heart failure/biventricular failure:

- Swelling in the legs (oedema).
- The oedema may lead to dry skin on the lower part of the legs due to pressure from inside the tissue. There may also be an eczema-type rash which can be complicated by ulcers that do not heal (venous leg ulcers).
- Possible accumulation of fluid in the abdominal cavity and organs, especially the liver. The organs swell and the abdominal wall might expand.

Classification of heart failure

The severity of heart failure is scored according to the 'New York Heart Failure Association' (NYHA) classification system. Within this system, the patient's symptom profile is used to determine which classification they fit into, the least severe being classification I and the more severe being classification IV. In some instances, the person can be positioned between two classifications. A more descriptive account of the NYHA classification system is presented in the following:

- **Class I:** the person has symptoms of dyspnoea with more than ordinary activity
- **Class II:** the person has these symptoms with ordinary activity
- **Class III:** there are symptoms of dyspnoea with minimal activity, so the condition is increasing in its severity
- **Class IV:** the person is experiencing symptoms at rest so is most affected by the disease.

(The Criteria Committee of the New York Heart Association, 1994)

Outlook

Heart failure is progressive with gradual deterioration which may be interspersed by acute episodes, but treatment can often slow the progression of the illness and substantially increase the patient's quality of life.

Management

The aim of management is to maintain the best quality of life for as long as possible. Optimum management will require a multidisciplinary approach. Inevitably, the condition will deteriorate and at some future point palliative care may be indicated. Where possible, reversible causes should be managed appropriately. It is important to (a) reduce the work of the heart and (b) to support the failing heart to pump as effectively as possible. These can be achieved by a combination of lifestyle changes and drug therapy (SIGN 95, 2007).

Lifestyle changes include:

- Daily weight – if >1.5 kg in 2 days consult general practitioner (GP)/specialist nurse
- Dietary changes
  — Reduced calorie intake if overweight
  — Limit saturated fat and cholesterol
  — Salt restriction
  — Avoidance of grapefruit and cranberry juice may be necessary to avoid certain drug interactions
- Smoking cessation
- Low-intensity physical exercise in stable heart failure (HF)
- Restrict alcohol intake to recommended limits
- Sexual activity – patients on nitrates should not take phosphodiesterase type 5 inhibitors [e.g. sildenafil (Viagra) or tadalafil (Cialis)]. This may lead to profound hypotension.

It may be necessary to limit fluid intake but this should only be undertaken on the advice of your physician/specialist nurse.

Drug therapy may include:

- Angiotensin converting enzyme (ACE) inhibitors
- β blockers
- Angiotensin II receptor blockers
- Aldosterone antagonists
- Diuretics
- Digoxin
- Nitrates
- Immunisations for pneumococcal and annual flu vaccine.

It is important that patients are regularly assessed by appropriate health-care personnel.

Patients who no longer respond to lifestyle changes and drug therapy should be referred to a specialist centre for assessment for cardiac transplantation.

Summary

The activity of breathing involves a number of different body systems. Whilst some reserve capacity is lost with ageing, growing older does not inevitably mean increasing breathlessness and an inability to engage in even vigorous and strenuous activities. However, problems with breathing can be very life-limiting and restrictive.

Pneumonia is a serious and life-threatening condition in older people. Similarly, influenza is highly contagious and very dangerous when contracted by older adults. Heart failure is a complex syndrome that invariably restricts a person's activities of living. Breathlessness is a key feature of heart failure.

References and further reading

Balicer, R.D., Huerta, M., Levy, Y., Davidovitch, N. and Grotto, I. 2005. Influenza outbreak control in confined settings. Emergency Infectious Diseases 11(4), 579–583.

Banning, M. 2005. Influenza: incidence, symptoms and treatment. British Journal of Nursing 14(22), 1192–1196.

Cleland, J.G.F., Swedberg, K., Follath, F., et al. 2003. The EuroHeart Failure survey programme—a survey on the quality of care among patients with heart failure in Europe: Part 1: patient Characteristics and diagnosis. European Heart Journal 24(5), 442–463.

Cowie, M.R., Fox, K., Wood, D.A., et al. 2002. Hospitalization of patients with heart failure. A population-based study. European Heart Journal 23(11), 877–885.

Davis, R.C., Hobbs, F.D.R. and Lip, G.Y.H. 2000. ABC of heart failure, history and epidemiology. British Medical Journal 320, 39–42.

De Geest, S., Scheurweghs, L., Reynders, I., et al. 2003. Differences in psychosocial and behavioural profiles between heart failure patients admitted to cardiology and geriatric wards. European Journal of Heart Failure 5(4), 557–567.

De Geest, S., Steelman, E., Leventhal, M.E., et al. 2004. Complexity in caring for an ageing heart failure population: concomitant chronic conditions and age related impairments. European Journal of Cardiovascular Nursing 3, 263–270.

De Martinis, M. and Timiras, P. 2003. The pulmonary respiration, hematopoiesis and erythrocytes. In Timiras, P. (Ed). Physiological Basis of Aging and Geriatrics. 3rd ed. CRC Press, Boca Raton, FL.

Dyer, C.A.E. and Stockley, R.A. 2006. The aging lung. Reviews in Clinical Gerontology 16, 99–111.

Evans, M., Prout, H., Prior, L., Tapper-Jones, L. and Butler, C. 2007. A qualitative study of lay beliefs about influenza immunisation in older people. British Journal of General Practice 57(538), 352–358.

Francis, C. 2006. Respiratory Care. Blackwell Publishing, Oxford.

Heath, H. and Schofield, I. 1999. Healthy Ageing: Nursing Older People. Mosby, London.

Jaarsma, T., Stromberg, A., De Geest, S., et al. 2006. Heart failure management programmes in Europe. European Journal of Cardiovascular Nursing 5, 197–205.

Jevon, P. and Ewens, B. 2001. Assessment of a breathless patient. Nursing Standard 15(16), 48–53.

Lueckenotte, A.G. 2000. Gerontologic Nursing. 2nd ed. Mosby, St. Louis, MO.

Mangtani, P., Breeze, E., Stirling, S., Hanciles, S., Kovats, S. and Fletcher, A. 2006. Cross-sectional survey of older peoples' views related to influenza vaccine uptake. BMC Public Health 6, 249. Doi:10.1186/1471-2458-6-249.

Mauk, K.L. 2006. Gerontological Nursing: Competencies for Care. Jones and Bartlett Publishers, Sudbury, MA.

Meiner, S.E. and Lueckenotte, A.G. 2006. Gerontologic Nursing. 3rd ed. Mosby Elsevier, St. Louis, MO.

Nair, M. and Peate, I. (Eds). 2009. Fundamentals of Applied Pathophysiology. An Essential Guide for Nursing Students. Wiley-Blackwell, Chichester, p. 219, figure 9.4.

NICE. 2003. Chronic Heart Failure. National Clinical Guideline for Diagnosis and Management in Primary and Secondary Care. CG5. Royal College of Physicians, London.

Petersen, S., Rayner, M. and Wolstenholme, J. 2002. Coronary Heart Disease Statistics: Heart Failure Supplement. British Heart Foundation Health Promotion Research Group, Oxford, pp. 1–36.

Quinn, M., Babb, P., Brock, A., Kirby, L. and Jones, J. 2001. Cancer Trends in England and Wales 1950–1999. The Stationery Office, London.

Roach, S. 2001. Introductory Gerontological Nursing. Lippincott, Philadelphia, PA.

Seeley, R.R., Stephens, T.D. and Tate, P. 2003. Anatomy and Physiology. 6th ed. McGraw Hill, London.

Sheahan, S.L. and Musialowski, R. 2001. Clinical implications of respiratory system changes in aging. Journal of Gerontological Nursing 27(5), 26–34.

SIGN. 2007. Management of Chronic Heart Failure. A National Clinical Guideline (95). Scottish Intercollegiate Guidelines Network, Edinburgh.

The Criteria Committee of the New York Heart Association. 1994. Nomenclature and Criteria for Diagnosis of Diseases of the Heart and Great Vessels. 9th ed. Little, Brown and Co., Boston, MA, pp. 253–256.

Tortora, G. and Derrickson, B. 2007. Introduction to the Human Body: The Essentials of Anatomy and Physiology. 7th ed. John Wiley & Sons, New York, NY, pp. 371 and 450, figures 15.5a,b and 18.4.

Tortora, G.J. and Derrickson, B.H. 2009. Principles of Anatomy and Physiology. 12th ed. John Wiley & Sons, New Jersey.

Tortora, G.J. and Grabowski, S.R. 2004. Introduction to the Human Body. The Essentials of Anatomy and Physiology. 6th ed. John Wiley & Sons, New Jersey.

Watson, E.D. 2009. The Partner's Experience of Heart Failure: Accommodating the Unanticipated. Unpublished Ph.D. Thesis. University of Dundee, Dundee, Scotland.

Waugh, A. and Grant, A. 2006. Ross and Wilson's Anatomy and Physiology in Health and Illness. Churchill Livingstone Elsevier, Edinburgh.

While, A., George, C. and Murgatroyd, B. 2005. Promoting influenza vaccination in older people: rationale and reality. British Journal of Community Nursing 10(9), 427–430.

Useful websites

Heart Failure Online. http://www.heartfailure.org/.

Medline Plus: Heart Failure. http://www.nlm.nih.gov/medlineplus/ency/article/000158.htm.

Chapter 6

Eating and Drinking

Aims

After reading this chapter you will be able to examine the activity of eating and drinking in older adults.

Learning Outcomes

After completion of this chapter you will be able to:

- Describe the normal structure and function of the gastrointestinal system and the associated structures
- Conduct a comprehensive patient nutritional assessment using appropriate tools
- Detail the changes in the above systems that are associated with ageing
- Discuss the presentation and management of some common health problems related to the above systems that occur in older adults.

Introduction

We will begin this chapter with an overview of the normal anatomy and physiology of the gastrointestinal system (GI). It will include a summary of the dietary and fluid requirements for older people. After this we will then go on to examine changes within the GI system associated with ageing, discussing the effects ageing has on the older person's ability to digest, absorb and eliminate food. Compensatory mechanisms such as the decreased speed of food passing through the small intestine (which occurs to compensate for the normal ageing process of flattening of the microvilli), reducing the risk of older adults becoming undernourished will be discussed.

We will then go on to consider how the health-care professional conducts a nutritional assessment. Assessment of bowel function will also be discussed. The common health

The Physiological Effects of Ageing: Implications for Nursing Practice, First Edition
© Alistair Farley, Ella McLafferty and Charles Hendry
Published 2011 by Blackwell Publishing Ltd

conditions of constipation and malnutrition in older adults will be discussed, including the nutritional support older patients require both in the community and in hospital settings. We will conclude with an examination of the nursing interventions that are required for older adults to attain and maintain a good nutritional status.

Normal structure and function

The GI, or digestive, system consists of the alimentary canal and a number of accessory organs. These include the liver, pancreas, gall bladder, teeth and the salivary glands. This system allows the body to take in nutrients in order to supply the cells with the 'building blocks' for metabolism and to excrete the remaining residue.

Activity

List the body's main nutrients and describe their functions within body cells. Identify good sources of the above nutrients for older adults.

Everyone must eat a varied diet in order to ensure that they are adequately supplied with all the necessary nutrients to maintain health. We need the right balance of nutrients for work, growth and repair. Exactly what constitutes the 'right' balance varies across the lifespan.

In the form in which we eat most of the food is much too big to cross cell membranes, so it must first be broken down into smaller units. This is achieved both mechanically and chemically within the GI system. General functions of the digestive system are outlined in Table 6.1.

The digestive system is a long, hollow, muscular tube ($\sim$9 m) extending from the mouth to the anus.

Table 6.1   General functions of the digestive system.

Ingestion	The action of taking food in, that is, eating. It consists of biting, chewing and swallowing for solids, and swallowing for liquids
Peristalsis	The movement of foodstuffs through the alimentary canal by involuntary muscular contractions
Digestion	The mechanical and chemical breakdown of ingested food into simpler sub-units
Absorption	The movement of nutrients through the lining of the alimentary canal into the blood and lymphatic system
Elimination	The excretion of indigestible residue from the body, that is, defaecation

The mouth

The mouth (also known as the oral or buccal cavity) is bordered by lips, cheeks, a hard and soft palate, a muscular floor and the oro-pharynx. It contains a highly muscular tongue, taste buds, salivary glands and teeth. Humans have two sets of teeth during their lifetime – a temporary set during childhood and a permanent set during adulthood. The mouth has several functions which are listed in Table 6.2.

 Revision Point

Three pairs of salivary glands, which produce saliva, open into the mouth. Name these glands, state their position and where they open into the mouth.

Saliva is largely made up from water (99%) which helps to moisten food. This process helps with taste; the taste buds can only be stimulated by chemical substances that are in solution and have therefore been dissolved in the saliva (Waugh and Grant, 2006). Mucus within saliva aids lubrication of food which enhances swallowing. Swallowing in the absence of adequate volumes of saliva becomes very difficult. The enzyme lysozyme contained within saliva helps to kill bacteria within the mouth. The other enzyme, salivary amylase, begins the chemical breakdown of complex sugars and starch to the disaccharide maltose (Seeley et al., 2003). Saliva has a typical pH of 6.7 which makes it slightly acidic. Sympathetic stimulation of the salivary glands inhibits saliva secretion during stressful moments, resulting in a dry mouth. When stimulated by the parasympathetic division of the ANS, more saliva is secreted to aid with digestion of foodstuffs. Saliva is secreted in anticipation of eating where the mere thought or sight of food will stimulate its release. This release is continued when food enters the mouth and the process of digestion begins.

Once swallowed, food passes through the pharynx and is propelled down the oesophagus by peristaltic action. Peristalsis is the rhythmic contraction of smooth muscles which propels foodstuffs through the digestive tract. The oesophagus passes through the diaphragm and opens into the stomach at the cardiac sphincter.

 Revision Point

Identify the different structures and organs that make up the digestive system.

Table 6.2   Functions of the mouth.

Mechanical digestion of food
Chemical digestion of food
Taste
Swallowing
Speech

The stomach

The stomach is a 'J' shaped organ situated just below the diaphragm. It is divided into four main regions – cardiac region, fundus, body and pylorus. The stomach has a lesser curvature and a greater curvature which provide attachments for folds of the peritoneum.

The gastric wall has three layers of muscle – an outer longitudinal layer, a middle circular layer and an inner oblique layer. These allow for the churning action of the stomach moving food forwards and backwards, a process which aids in the breakdown of food.

The sub-mucosa and mucosa are thrown into folds known as rugae, which greatly increase the surface area for secretion of digestive juices and allow for considerable distension following ingestion of a meal. The gastric mucosa contains deep gastric pits which are the openings for the gastric glands. Cells found within the gastric pits include surface mucous cells which secrete mucus, mucous neck cells which also secrete mucus, parietal cells which secrete hydrochloric acid (HCl) and intrinsic factor (necessary for the absorption of vitamin B_{12}), endocrine cells which secrete the hormone gastrin and finally chief cells which secrete the enzyme pepsinogen.

Mucus protects the lining of the stomach from the actions of gastric juice. HCl acidifies food, stops the chemical breakdown of starch to maltose and converts inactive pepsinogen to the active form pepsin, which breaks down proteins to smaller units called polypeptides (hence beginning the chemical digestion of proteins). Pepsins work best at a pH of 1.5–3.5. Intrinsic factor combines with vitamin B_{12} to allow for its absorption. The hormone gastrin stimulates gastric glands to release gastric juice.

The contents of gastric juice can be found in Table 6.3.

The functions of the stomach can be found in Table 6.4.

Table 6.3 Constituents of gastric juice.

Water
Mucus
Mineral salts
Hydrochloric acid (HCl) – pH 1–3
Intrinsic factor
Pepsinogen

Table 6.4 Functions of the stomach.

Reservoir for food
Protection through action of HCl
Mechanical digestion (churning of muscles)
Chemical digestion through action of enzymes
Limited absorption of water, alcohol, glucose and some drugs

The mechanical and chemical digestion which occurs in the stomach results in a semi-fluid liquid called chyme. This liquid can remain in the stomach for many hours before eventually being transported into the duodenum.

The small intestine

Chyme passes through the pyloric sphincter into the small intestine, a long tube 7 m in length which lies coiled up in the abdominal cavity. The small intestine is divided into three parts – duodenum, jejunum and ileum.

The duodenum, which is the first part of the small intestine, receives secretions from the pancreas (pancreatic juice) and the gall bladder (bile), both of which release these secretions into the duodenum via the hepatopancreatic ampulla (also known as the ampulla of Vater). The ileum of the small intestine terminates at the ileo-caecal valve leading to the large intestine or colon.

The mucous membrane lining of the small intestine is designed to greatly increase its surface area. It achieves this by the presence of circular folds, villi and microvilli (Figure 6.1). The circular folds around the intestine enhance absorption by causing the chyme to spiral through the intestine rather than moving through in a straight line. This slows the whole process thereby enhancing digestion and absorption. Villi are finger-like projections of the mucosa, richly supplied with blood capillaries, into which the products of digestion

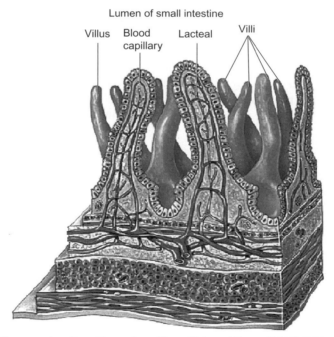

Figure 6.1 Diagram of a villus. (Reproduced from Nair and Peate (2009). With permission from John Wiley & Sons.)

Table 6.5   Hormones necessary for chemical digestion of food.

Hormone	Released from	Actions
Gastrin	Stomach	Stimulates gastric glands to produce gastric juice
Enteric gastrin	Small intestine	Continued stimulation of gastric glands
Gastric inhibiting peptide	Small intestine	Stops production of gastric juice
Secretin	Small intestine	Stimulates release of intestinal juice and pancreatic juice
Cholecystokinin	Small intestine	Stimulates release of pancreatic juice and bile

are absorbed. They also contain a lymphatic vessel or central lacteal into which fatty acids, glycerol and fat-soluble vitamins are absorbed. The microvilli project from the apex of the villi and increase the overall surface area available for absorption. They form a fuzzy line at the apical surface of the villi known as the brush border.

The chyme within the small intestine undergoes chemical digestion from (i) intestinal juice from the intestinal glands, (ii) pancreatic juice secreted by acinar cells in the pancreas and (iii) bile produced by the liver and stored and concentrated in the gall bladder until required.

Tables 6.5 and 6.6 list the hormones and enzymes necessary for the chemical digestion of food.

In the process of chemical digestion, carbohydrates, fats and proteins are broken down to their smallest units of mainly glucose, fatty acids and glycerol and amino acids. This renders them small enough to be absorbed through the gut wall. Most of the absorption of nutrients from the digestive tract takes place through the wall of the small intestine into the blood and lymphatic system.

Absorption of nutrients in small intestine

Glucose absorption

- Monosaccharides enter the epithelial cells of a villus (through the microvilli)
- They leave the epithelial cells to enter a blood capillary within a villus
- They are then transported to the liver via the hepatic portal vein.

Protein absorption

- Amino acids enter the epithelial cells of a villus
- They leave the cells to enter a blood capillary within a villus
- They too are then transported to the liver via the hepatic portal vein.

Table 6.6 Enzymes necessary for chemical digestion of food.

Enzyme	Released from	Action
Salivary amylase	Mouth	Breaks down starch to maltose
Pepsin	Stomach	Converts proteins to peptides
Rennin	Stomach in infants	Curdles (solidifies) milk
Enterokinase	Small intestine	Converts inactive trypsinogen to active trypsin
Peptidases	Small intestine	Convert peptides to amino acids
Lipase	Small intestine	Converts lipids to fatty acids and glycerol
Sucrase	Small intestine	Converts sucrose to glucose and fructose
Maltase	Small intestine	Converts maltose to glucose
Lactase	Small intestine	Converts lactose to glucose and galactose
Trypsinogen	Pancreas	Converted to trypsin by enterokinase. Trypsin converts polypeptides to peptides
Chymotrypsinogen	Pancreas	Converted to active chymotrypsin by trypsin. Chymotrypsin converts polypeptides to peptides
Carboxypeptidase	Pancreas	Converts polypeptides to peptides and amino acids
Pancreatic amylase	Pancreas	Converts polysaccharides to disaccharides
Pancreatic lipase	Pancreas	Converts lipids to fatty acids and glycerol
Ribonuclease	Pancreas	Converts RNA nucleotides to pentoses and nitrogenous bases
Deoxyribonuclease	Pancreas	Converts DNA nucleotides to pentoses and nitrogenous bases
Bile	Gall bladder	Emulsifies fat droplets into smaller particles

Fat absorption

- Bile salts form aggregates called micelles in the small intestine
- Fatty acids and glycerol dissolve into these micelles in the small intestine
- Micelles now come into contact with the surface of the epithelial cells
- Fatty acids and glycerol diffuse into the cells
- Micelles stay behind in the chyme
- Once inside the epithelial cells, the fatty acids and glycerol recombine to form triglycerides (fats)
- Triglycerides unite with cholesterol and become coated with proteins and are now known as chylomicrons
- Chylomicrons leave the epithelial cells and enter the lacteal of a villus
- They are then transported in lymphatic vessels as chyle (this is lymph fluid which is high in lipids)

- The chyle is transported to the thoracic duct and enters the bloodstream at the left subclavian vein
- The fats eventually enter the liver via the hepatic artery.

Activity

Identify which nutrients are absorbed directly into the blood and which are initially absorbed into the lymphatic system. Describe how these nutrients reach the liver once they have been absorbed.

The large intestine

The large intestine extends from the ileo-caecal valve to the anus through which digestive residue is eliminated as faeces. It lies in an arch around the abdominal cavity, surrounding the small intestine. The functions of the large intestine can be seen in Table 6.7.

 Revision Point

Arrange the following parts of the large intestine in the correct order:

- Rectum
- Caecum
- Hepatic flexure
- Ascending colon
- Anal canal
- Sigmoid colon
- Transverse colon
- Descending colon
- Splenic flexure.

Table 6.7 Functions of the large intestine.

Absorbs water (consolidation of faeces)
Absorbs some electrolytes
Absorbs vitamin K – synthesised from bacteria in the large bowel
Secretes mucus to lubricate faeces
Temporary storage of indigestible foodstuffs until they are eliminated from the body
Bacteria cause the fermentation of undigested food residues with the production of gases – hydrogen, carbon dioxide and methane
Bacteria in the large intestine also synthesise vitamin K and folic acid – a valuable source of these vitamins within the body

As previously identified, the ileum of the small intestine terminates at the ileo-caecal valve leading to the large intestine. Longitudinal muscles of the large intestine are gathered into three bands known as taeniae coli. Contraction of these bands gathers the colon into a series of pouches known as haustra, which give the colon its puckered appearance.

Movement of the contents within the large intestine occurs via three mechanisms. Haustral churning occurs whilst they receive faecal contents as the haustra remain relaxed and distended. As the distension grows, a critical point is reached when the haustrum contracts and squeezes the contents into the next haustrum. Peristalsis also occurs in the ascending colon of the large intestine at the rate of 3–12 contractions every minute. Finally, mass movements (mass peristalsis) also occur from the middle of the transverse colon to the descending colon which quickly drives colonic contents into the rectum. Mass movements occur 3–4 times every day usually during or after eating (Seeley et al., 2003; Tortora, 2005). It should be noted that mass movements are said to be most common shortly after breakfast (Seeley et al., 2003).

 Point for Practice

How would you incorporate the above knowledge into a plan of care for older adults in a residential, nursing home or hospital setting?

When the colon's contents are moved into the descending colon and rectum, stretch receptors stimulate nerves initiating a reflex action of contraction of the rectum and relaxation of the internal sphincter. The external sphincter is voluntarily controlled until a suitable time and place is found in order for defaecation to occur.

Although chemical digestion does not take place in the large intestine, it has a very important function in relation to the absorption of water. Up to 7 l of digestive juices are secreted by the digestive system every day. Without re-absorption of the water and salts from these juices, dehydration would soon result.

 Revision Point

Compare the composition of the contents of the small bowel at the ileo-caecal junction with that in the rectum.

The liver

Although not specifically part of the digestive system, the liver has many functions associated with digestion and nutrients.

The liver is the largest gland in the body weighing about 1.4 kg in an average adult (Tortora, 2005). It lies in the right upper abdomen just under the diaphragm. Much of the liver is shielded by the ribs. It is roughly triangular shaped and is divided into two main lobes (Tortora, 2005). The lobes consist of smaller portions known as lobules in which cells are arranged in columns like spokes of a wheel. Between the columns of cells, the blood flows through incomplete capillaries called sinusoids which allow the blood to come in contact with liver cells. The lobules are made up from specialised epithelial cells called hepatocytes. Amongst other functions, hepatocytes are involved with the formation and secretion of bile. Hepatocytes are also associated with protein synthesis and can store glycogen, vitamins (A, B_{12}, D, E and K), copper and iron (Seeley et al., 2003; Tortora, 2005). Blood vessels, ducts and nerves enter and leave the liver at the portal fissure on its inferior surface.

 Revision Point

1. The liver receives blood from two different vessels. Name these vessels and their origin. Differentiate between the contents of blood carried in the vessels.
2. Trace the passage of bile from its manufacture in the lobules to its entry into the duodenum.
3. Name the substances which the liver
   - Stores
   - Manufactures
   - Detoxifies.

The gall bladder

The gall bladder is located on the inferior surface of the liver and is a pear-shaped sac. It stores, concentrates and excretes bile which is produced in the liver. Bile consists of water, mineral salts, bile salts, bile pigments and cholesterol. The pH of bile is between 7 and 9, making it slightly alkaline. Bile is involved in the chemical digestion of foodstuffs through the action of its bile salts where it emulsifies fat globules into smaller droplets. This action takes place within the small intestine. Bile salts also make cholesterol and fatty acids soluble, enabling these and the fat-soluble vitamins (A, D, E and K) to be easily absorbed.

The pancreas

The pancreas is situated behind the greater curvature of the stomach and consists of a head, body and tail. It secretes pancreatic juice (exocrine function) which leaves the pancreas in ducts that join to form the main pancreatic duct. This joins with the common bile duct and empties into the duodenum at the hepatopancreatic ampulla. Pancreatic juice consists of water, mineral salts, sodium bicarbonate and the enzymes trypsinogen, chymotrypsinogen, pancreatic amylase and pancreatic lipase.

Sodium bicarbonate is alkaline and therefore neutralises acidic chyme in the small intestine and helps to create an environment conducive for digestive enzyme functioning. The pancreas is involved in the chemical digestion of foodstuffs through the action of its enzymes. Refer to Table 6.6 naming the enzymes necessary for chemical digestion of food.

The pancreas also has an endocrine function where it secretes and releases hormones including insulin, in relation to blood glucose homeostasis.

Ageing changes in the digestive system

There are few alterations in GI function associated with ageing, although cellular changes do occur involving secretory activity and motility of the major structures. These cellular changes are similar to that elsewhere in the body and despite these physiological alterations, GI function is usually maintained in line with body needs.

As already discussed, the major function of the GI system is to provide nutrition to the body. This is achieved by the mechanical and chemical processes of digestion, absorption, storage or movement of foods and excretion of unabsorbed elements.

The liver is the organ most severely affected by ageing. Bile formation stays quite stable in healthy individuals well into old age. The detoxification of both therapeutic and recreational drugs is progressively restricted with advancing age.

Many people lose their teeth by the age of 40 as a result of periodontal disease or infection (Christiansen and Grzybowski, 1999). However, today, older people are more likely to retain more of their natural dentition. This improvement is related to changing attitudes associated with loss of teeth in old age, improved health education and knowledge about dental care, increased use of fluoride (e.g. in water and in toothpaste) and increased availability of dental services (Matteson et al., 1997).

However, the teeth do undergo characteristic changes associated with ageing. They often acquire a yellowish-brown discolouration from staining caused by pigments found in beverages, tobacco and foodstuffs. The presence and action of oral bacteria also contribute to this discolouration (Timiras, 2003).

Tooth enamel becomes less permeable and more brittle, chipping and fracturing easily (Christiansen and Grzybowski, 1999). Within the pulp cavity, nerves degenerate and atherosclerosis affects the tiny blood vessels supplying the teeth, causing the teeth to become brittle (Roach, 2001).

Chewing surfaces on the teeth wear down so that they no longer match well when eating food. The grinding and chewing of food by the teeth results in beneficial chewing stress which helps to maintain bone health in the jaw. Loss or removal of teeth results in a reduction in this beneficial process. Bone loss in the jaw, associated with ageing (osteoporosis), contributes to the loosening of otherwise healthy teeth (Christiansen and Grzybowski, 1999; Timiras, 2003). Despite these changes, loss of teeth is not inevitable (Roach, 2001).

Recession of the gingivae occurs in all older people (Timiras, 2003) and results in an appearance of longer teeth than before, giving rise to the expression of being long in the tooth (Christiansen and Grzybowski, 1999). As gums recede, it becomes more difficult to maintain well-fitted dentures.

Older people are less likely to develop new dental caries. However, loss of interest in dental hygiene and loss of manual dexterity may lead to the build up of plaque and the subsequent formation of dental caries in the older adult (Timiras, 2003).

Structures on the tongue called papillae, many of which contain taste buds, atrophy with age. This atrophy is associated with the loss of taste. The ability to both detect and identify food flavours – salt, sweet, sour and bitter – decreases with age. There may be some increase in taste threshold for salt and sugars, causing bitter tastes to predominate (Deems et al., 1991). Brownie (2006) also states that sweet and salty taste decline first so that food begins to taste sour and bitter. However, Matteson et al. (1997) suggest that the sensation of taste only modestly decreases with age.

Secretions of the salivary glands reduce with age (Matteson et al., 1997), leading to a dry mouth which sometimes makes swallowing difficult (Roach, 2001). Heath and Schofield (1999) state that saliva production can be decreased as a consequence of a reduction in secretory cells by as much as 25% as they are replaced by fibrous or fatty tissue. They go on to claim that from the age of 50, salivary amylase is reduced and this impedes digestion of complex carbohydrates.

Thirst regulation is often affected making dehydration a prime risk among older adults (Lueckenotte, 2000). The sensation of thirst also changes with age (Mack et al., 1994). In older adults, a lack of sensation when the body is becoming fluid depleted may be due to a reduction in hypothalamic awareness of a change in body fluid status. As a result, an older adult can become dehydrated and not realise nor respond to this condition physiologically. Older adults can therefore lose fluids without stimulating the thirst response (Kenney and Chiu, 2001). As such, older adults may not request fluids to drink as they may not feel thirsty.

In the oesophagus, reflex actions triggered by the presence of food drive the contents downwards, through smooth muscle contractions known as peristalsis. These processes require a correctly timed contraction and relaxation order. However, this order can be affected with age, as it may become desynchronised resulting in swallowing difficulties (Timiras, 2003).

By the age of 64, the gastric mucosa has usually undergone some degree of atrophy (Christiansen and Grzybowski, 1999). In healthy older people, the mucosal cells in the stomach and small intestine atrophy and the production of hydrochloric acid is reduced (Roach, 2001; Timiras, 2003). This reduction in acid also decreases the rate of enzyme release such as pepsin which may result in difficulties digesting protein-rich foods (Timiras, 2003). The reduction of the mucous protective layer in the stomach increases the risk of attack from HCl and protein digesting enzymes which can then readily destroy the exposed mucosal cells (Timiras, 2003). A reduction in prostaglandin production associated with ageing contributes to the loss of the gastric mucosa. Prostaglandins enhance bicarbonate release which assists with protection of the mucosa from acid and digestive enzymes. This protective cover is reduced when less bicarbonate is produced associated with a reduction in prostaglandin levels. All of this increases the likelihood of gastritis and peptic ulceration (Timiras, 2003).

Associated with ageing is a decreased elasticity of the stomach, resulting in a reduction in accommodation of food. Gastric emptying is also slower with advancing age (Meiner and Lueckenotte, 2006). Production of intrinsic factor also decreases which is necessary for the absorption of vitamin B_{12}. This can increase the incidence of pernicious anaemia in the older adult (Roach, 2001).

Many factors affect the absorption of digested foodstuffs, including the speed of passage of food through the digestive tract, any alterations to the absorptive surfaces of the digestive tract, the blood supply to the digestive system and the effectiveness of the transport mechanism involved. Dextrose and xylose are absorbed more slowly and fat absorption also tends to be slower in older people (Heath and Schofield, 1999). This can contribute to the feeling of fullness and a resulting reduction in appetite. Absorption of calcium, iron and vitamins B_1 and B_2 decreases with age. The number of villi and microvilli in the small intestine reduce with age. They also decrease in height and increase in breadth, resulting in a significant reduction in mucosal surface area (Matteson et al., 1997). However, because there are more than 4 million villi/microvilli, this reduction in numbers and size does not significantly affect the absorption of most nutrients (Roach, 2001).

Changes in the large bowel include loss of mucosa, excess connective tissue and vascular changes which are largely due to atherosclerosis. The blood vessels supplying the colon may become tortuous which can impede the flow of blood to the colon (Matteson et al., 1997). There is a decrease in overall muscle strength and a reduction in peristaltic actions (Matteson et al., 1997; Roach, 2001). Decreased motility can contribute to the development of constipation which may also be linked to a diet lacking in fibre and fluids or to a lack of exercise (Roach, 2001; Timiras, 2003). There is an increase in the prevalence of diverticula in people over the age of 50, with increasing incidence thereafter. As stated, the presence of diverticulitis is common but it is not entirely clear whether this is related only to age or as a result of a lack of dietary fibre linked to constipation (Roach, 2001).

Frequency of defaecation remains the same after the age of 60 as compared to before 60. However, the volume of distension in the rectum necessary to stimulate the desire to defaecate is larger in older people.

With advancing age, the pancreas may become smaller and harder due to increasing fibrosis. Accumulation of lipofuscin (a pigment associated with ageing) can be noted which is also found on other organs such as the kidneys, heart and liver (Matteson et al., 1997; Timiras, 2003). Only one-tenth of the pancreas is required for normal digestion (Timiras, 2003), therefore the pancreas can be seen to have a large reserve capacity (Matteson et al., 1997). The total volume of secretions from the pancreas reduces after the fourth decade and enzyme release also reduces with age (Meiner and Lueckenotte, 2006). However, despite these changes, the production of bicarbonate, amylase and trypsin remains adequate to meet body demands (Matteson et al., 1997).

Ageing does not appear to affect the gall bladder or bile ducts. However, gallstones are more likely to occur with advancing age (Meiner and Lueckenotte, 2006).

After the age of 70, the liver decreases in size and secretes less enzymes than before. The reduction in size of the liver decreases the space available for storage of nutrients such as proteins, vitamins, minerals and glycogen. The reduction in hepatic enzymes interferes with metabolism and makes the detoxification of drugs more difficult (Roach, 2001).

According to Matteson et al. (1997), the metabolism of drugs may be reduced by as much as 30% from adulthood to old age. There is also a decrease in the production of bile and cholesterol associated with ageing.

The number of hepatocytes in the lobules decline with age. Protein synthesis within these hepatocytes is also reduced. This reduction in protein synthesis is associated with a decrease in enzymatic activity (Christiansen and Grzybowski, 1999). However, changes are usually quite minor and the liver has enough reserve capacity to accommodate these changes. Hepatic cells regenerate throughout life, but the regeneration slows as we age (Timiras, 2003).

Oral hygiene

The aim of oral hygiene is to keep the oral mucosa clean, moist and soft and to prevent the lips from cracking. Any food debris and dental plaque should be removed from the mouth and teeth. These actions should ensure a comfortable mouth and prevent halitosis. Good fluid intake will enhance these actions.

Older people require to have their mouths checked (assessed) and cleaned whether they have their natural teeth or otherwise. This assessment should form part of any admission procedure and should be repeated as often as is necessary. Many older adults living at home will follow a regular pattern of oral hygiene familiar to them. If removed from their home environment for whatever reasons, they should be enabled to follow their typical oral hygiene care patterns for as long as possible.

It should be recognised that many older care settings may not have adequate facilities for the maintenance of privacy and dignity when engaged in personal oral hygiene. Open style ward areas and shared bathroom facilities, inadequate lighting and fixtures which are not easy to reach and use do not enhance or encourage the maintenance of self-care. Furthermore, fixed routines within health-care settings may present as a barrier to independence and actually promote dependence in the care setting (British Society for Disability and Oral Health (BSDH), 2000).

Adams (1996) claimed that nurses in clinical practice lacked relevant knowledge in relation to oral health problems. White (2000) went on to claim that poor clinical knowledge of oral health problems was directly a consequence of poor education relating to oral hygiene and oral health care in nurses preregistration undergraduate programmes. They go on to state that this educational deficit can negatively impact on oral health care needs of older patients.

The ageing process has to be taken into account when considering the oral health needs of older adults. Teeth become loose and increasingly fragile relating to loss of gum tissue. There are changes in tooth structure related to simple wear and tear. As a result of these changes, the teeth are more easily damaged. The sockets in which the upper teeth are housed lose bone tissue, resulting in the teeth becoming slack and easily dislodged. The production of saliva is reduced. Muscles involved in the chewing of food are in some instances, used less, partly in relation to the use of softer food which requires less chewing action. Muscle tone is therefore reduced and over time muscle wasting can become apparent. When the muscles involved in chewing food become atrophied, food remains in the mouth for longer than before. Winkley et al. (1993) suggests that this allows sugars to remain in the oral cavity for longer periods of time which adds to the risk of dental caries.

The taste of food is affected by the presence of plaque and debris in the mouth, which in turn can reduce a person's appetite and readiness to eat and drink. Without appropriate oral care, patients may develop dental and oral diseases, which can affect eating and drinking (Simons et al., 1999). Good oral health care therefore not only keeps the oral cavity clean and moist, it also helps to maintain appetite and enjoyment of food and drink, thus helping to encourage adequate nutritional and fluid intake.

Speech is affected by the condition of the oral cavity. Ill-fitting dentures and damaged teeth both influence the ability to speak clearly and pronounce words accurately. Infection and inflammation of the mouth also make it difficult for the individual to articulate their words and speak clearly. These conditions not only impact on the person's ability to communicate with health-care professionals, but also impact on the ability to communicate with friends and family. In turn, this can lead to a withdrawal from family and wider social circles leading to social isolation.

Plaque and debris in the mouth can lead to bad breath or halitosis. Jones (1998) suggested that halitosis affects an individual psychologically and that this condition can negatively influence relationships within the family. Good oral health can help with self-image and self-esteem and enhance general well-being in older adults (Holmes, 1996).

Assessment of oral health

Roberts (2000a) claims that there is little evidence to indicate that oral assessment is taking place in clinical practice. During a global assessment, an assessment of your patient's oral health status should also be included. An easy to use assessment tool is outlined below. This will allow for appropriate oral care interventions to be put into practice where necessary. During this assessment, advice in relation to improving oral health status can also be offered.

The following areas should be assessed:

- Teeth – identify for presence of plaque, debris and decay. If wearing dentures, are they well fitting?
- Mucous membranes and gums – identify any areas of redness, bleeding or evidence of ulceration
- Tongue – check for size, colour, dryness, cracks or blisters
- Saliva – quantity and quality
- Lips – evidence of cracking, blistering or peeling?
- Halitosis – presence or absence of?

(Adapted from Endacott et al., 2009, p. 82)

A simple, straightforward oral assessment should be completed on admission to a residential care setting (BSDH, 2000). Such an assessment will highlight any oral health problems and help in the planning of good oral care. The oral assessment should be included in the routine assessment by staff.

Nursing management of oral hygiene

There are a number of readily available products which can be used to help maintain good oral hygiene. The toothbrush is the most commonly used and should continue to be used unless the person has difficulties with manual dexterity. A toothbrush should be used to clean both gums and tongue of all patients, even if the person wears dentures. However, toothpaste should not be used to clean dentures as it may damage the denture surface (Clarke, 1993). If your patient is unable to clean their own teeth, the toothbrush remains the most effective means by which good oral hygiene is achieved. Health carers should therefore carry out this skill for them, using an appropriate toothbrush and toothpaste.

As a toothbrush, toothpaste and water are most widely used to maintain good oral hygiene at home, it seems appropriate that this practice should continue if admitted to a care setting (Roberts, 2000b).

The use of lemon and glycerine swabs is no longer recommended as a means to obtain good oral hygiene (Bowsher et al., 1999). The presence of lemon can lower the pH within the oral cavity, leading to a more acidic environment which can be harmful to an older person's teeth. They also dry out the oral mucosa.

Foam sticks can be used to help cleanse and moisten the oral mucosa (Thurgood, 1994). However, they are not effective if used to remove plaque from the teeth (Bowsher et al., 1999).

The older method of using a gloved finger and a gauze swab cannot be recommended as a means to achieve good oral hygiene. The dangers of being bitten far outweigh the effectiveness of this method. This method can also push debris into gaps between the person's teeth which if not removed can add to the risk of oral infection.

A variety of mouthwashes are available including chlorhexidine mouthwash which has been shown to be useful in the control of plaque and for its antibacterial and fungicidal properties (Curzio and MacCowan, 2000). Such a mouthwash may be of benefit if your patient finds it difficult in cleaning their own teeth due to manual dexterity problems. Xavier (2000) advises that chlorhexidine is a useful addition to other oral health-care measures.

Although thymol or glycothymol mouthwashes have an initial refreshing action when used, they do not have any lasting beneficial effects (Nicol et al., 2000) or any cleansing actions within the oral cavity (Rattenbury et al., 1999).

The use of a lip lubricant can help to prevent drying and cracking of an older person's lips.

The eating of fresh fruit and drinking of fruit juices is something to be encouraged whether the older adult is at home or within a care setting. These not only provide essential vitamins but they are also refreshing and help to relieve a dry mouth.

If a person has dentures, they should be encouraged to remove them after each meal and rinse them under running cold water in order to remove any loose debris. If they cannot do this for themselves, a member of staff should perform these actions. It is also advisable to remove dentures overnight as this allows saliva to act upon acids which may have built up on the oral mucosa which would not be exposed if the dentures remain in place. Once removed, they should be cleaned and stored in cold water. They should neither be left to dry out, nor should be cleaned and stored in hot water as the dentures may warp and therefore become ill fitting. If dentures do not fit properly, this affects speech, mastication and can lead to discomfort and pain.

Nutritional assessment

Health-care professionals with appropriate skills and training should be involved in screening for malnutrition and risk of malnutrition. Holmes (2008, p. 48) states that 'malnutrition means bad nutrition and can include deficiency, excess or imbalance of energy (calories), protein or other nutrients (vitamins and minerals) that adversely affects body function and outcome'. Malnutrition can therefore include both under-nutrition and over-nutrition. The major concern for older people is under-nutrition, which has been described as that which falls below what is necessary to sustain life and well-being.

All hospital inpatients and outpatients at their first clinic appointment should be screened for nutritional status. Screening should be incorporated into all nursing records for older people. This procedure should be repeated weekly for inpatients and where deemed necessary for outpatients. People in care homes should be screened on admission and again when there is clinical concern. Clinical concern is described as unintentional weight loss, fragile skin, poor wound healing, apathy, wasted muscles, poor appetite, altered taste sensation, impaired swallowing, altered bowel habit, loose fitting clothes or prolonged illness (NICE, 2006).

The following guidelines are recommended by NICE (2006) in relation to nutritional support. Interventions should be considered in people who are malnourished as defined by the following:

- A body mass index (BMI) of less than $18.5\,kg/m^2$
- Recent unintentional weight loss greater than 10%
- BMI of less than $20\,kg/m^2$ and recent unintentional weight loss greater than 5%.

They also state that nutritional support should be considered in people at risk of malnutrition including those who have eaten little or nothing for more than 5 days and/or people who have been identified as likely to eat little or nothing for 5 days or more. People with known poor absorptive capacity and/or high nutrient losses or those with increased nutritional needs from causes such as catabolism also require nutritional support.

Nutritional screening has been defined as a simple and rapid procedure that facilitates identification of nutritional risk (Green and Watson, 2005), whereas nutritional assessment is the determination of nutritional status using appropriate objective markers such as dietary intake, biochemical data, anthropometry and clinical condition (National Nursing Midwifery and Health Visiting Advisory Committee, 2002). Screening is the first step in nutritional assessment and should be incorporated into all nursing records for older people.

National Health Service Quality Improvement Scotland (NHSQIS, 2003) states that an assessment should include screening for malnutrition using a validated tool; however, they also state that clinical judgement may allow for the exclusion of some patients from the fuller screening.

Green and Watson (2005) carried out a detailed review of nutritional assessment and screening tools used by nurses. They found a wide range of tools available and in use and concluded that there needs to be greater emphasis upon the reliability and validity of these tools. They also state that adopting the use of screening tools such as the one produced by the British Association of Parenteral and Enteral Nutrition (BAPEN) may help standardise the approach to nutritional screening – Malnutrition Universal Screening Tool (MUST).

Bowling (2004, p. 13) defines nutritional screening as a means of 'identifying patients who are malnourished or at risk of becoming undernourished'. The MUST was produced by BAPEN as means of identifying patients who are at risk of becoming malnourished whether they are underweight or obese. It is acknowledged that the tool is not designed to identify specific vitamin or mineral deviancies (BAPEN, 2003).

The tool consists of a five-step approach which culminates in a score that estimates the patient's risk and can be viewed at the following web address: http://www.bapen.org .uk/musttoolkit.html.

The score is related to recommended actions although Bowling (2004) adds that this will need to be supported by a care plan. Brown et al. (2006) state that MUST has a fair/good to excellent inter rater reliability and is quick to complete.

Steps in calculating MUST score:

- Measure height and weight to get a BMI score
- Note the percentage of unplanned weight loss and score
- Establish acute disease effect and score
- Add scores from steps 1, 2 and 3 together to obtain overall risk of malnutrition
- Use management guidelines and/or local policy to develop care plan

Score of 0 = low risk

- Screening repeated weekly in hospital, monthly in care homes, annually in community

Score of 1 = medium risk

- Document dietary intake for 3 days
- If no improvement, follow local policy for clinical concern
- Repeat screening as before

Score of 2 or above = high risk

- Referral to dietician, nutritional support team or implementation of other local policy
- Patient's nutritional intake should be increased
- Care plan should be monitored and reviewed weekly in hospital, monthly in care homes and community.

Although the BMI is widely accepted as the Gold Standard indicator of malnutrition, its use may mask important weight changes in all patients which can result in a nutritional problem being overlooked. BMI may also be unreliable in the presence of conditions including oedema and ascites. If used as a single screening tool in such patients, unintentional weight loss may be missed. Furthermore, in older adults, reliable measurement of height can be difficult due to vertebral decompression, loss of muscle tone and postural changes (Harris and Haboubi, 2005).

However, the BMI omits to acknowledge the significance of age and metabolism which decreases with age. This is associated with a decrease in lean body mass which results in a reduction in calories required to maintain this mass. The outcome is a decrease in nutritional requirements for energy (Blechman and Gelb, 1999). Lean body mass declines by about 1% each year starting at the age of 55. This decline is a direct result of a reduction in overall activity. However, total body weight does not change as rapidly due to the increase in the proportion of body fat associated with ageing. However, if physical activity remains high, this reduction in lean body mass can be delayed.

As identified earlier, screening for malnutrition should be carried out on initial contact with health-care professionals and those identified at risk should be further assessed and evaluated using an appropriate and validated assessment tool. NHSQIS (2003) suggests that the following procedures should be followed in relation to Standard 2 (Assessment,

Screening and Care Planning) of their document Clinical Standards for Food, Fluid and Nutritional Care in Hospitals (2003).

> When a person is admitted to hospital, an assessment is carried out. Screening for risk of under-nutrition is undertaken, both on admission and on an ongoing basis. A care plan is developed, implemented and evaluated.
>
> *(Standard 2 statement, p. 26)*

Essential criteria associated with the Standard 2 statement (NHSQIS, 2003):

When a person is admitted to hospital as an inpatient, the following are identified and recorded within 1 day as part of the medical/nursing assessment:
- Height and weight
- Eating and drinking likes/dislikes
- Cultural/ethnic/religious requirements
- Social/environmental mealtime requirements
- Physical difficulties with eating and drinking
- The need for equipment to help with eating and drinking.

The initial assessment includes screening for risk of under-nutrition. This screening is carried out using a validated tool appropriate to the patient population and which includes criteria and scores that indicate action to be taken.

Repeat screenings are undertaken in accordance with clinical need and at a frequency determined by the outcome of the initial and subsequent screenings.

The outcome of the screening is recorded in the medical notes.

The assessment process identifies the need for referral to specialist services, for example dietetic, dental.

Patients have access to specialist services within agreed timescale and access should be available 7 days a week for urgent cases.

When a person is admitted to hospital, an assessment is carried out. Screening for risk of under-nutrition is taken, both on admission and on an ongoing basis. A care plan is developed, implemented and evaluated.

The multidisciplinary care plan is followed, reviewed and refined, and includes:
- Outcomes of the initial assessment
- Outcomes of the screening for risk of under-nutrition
- Frequency/dates for repeat screening
- Actions taken as a consequence of repeat screening.

The discharge plan is developed with the patient and, where appropriate, carers, and includes information about:
- The patient's nutritional status
- Special dietary requirements
- The arrangements made for any follow-up required on nutritional issues.

Desirable criteria associated with the Standard 2 statement (NHSQIS, 2003):

- Patients referred to the dietetic service are seen within 2 days.

The Mini Nutritional Assessment (MNA) is a screening and assessment tool specifically developed for older people in relation to malnutrition. This tool can be viewed at the following web address: http://www.mna-elderly.com/. The MNA has 96% sensitivity and 98% specificity and a predictive value of 97% which distinguishes patients by their adequate nutritional status (Wells and Dumbrell, 2006).

Answers to questions in relation to the screening section are assigned points and if the tabulated scores from the six items contained within this section add up to 11 points or less, then the patient may be malnourished and the health-care provider is urged to complete the second part of the form which entails a fuller nutritional assessment.

This tool has been validated only for older adults over 55 (Brown et al., 2006). The goals of nutritional assessment are:

- Establish baseline subjective and objective nutrition parameters
- Identify specific nutritional deficits
- Determine nutritional risk factors
- Establish nutritional needs
- Identify medical and psychosocial factors that may influence the prescription and administration of nutrition support (Lueckenotte, 2000).

Common GI problems associated with ageing

Under-nutrition in older people

Weight loss in older people should not be ignored as it can be a sign of clinical disease. Weight loss due to voluntary or involuntary causes in older adults has been associated with mortality (Wells and Dumbrell, 2006). Early identification, assessment and treatment of weight loss and nutritional deficiencies can improve health status and quality of life in older adults. However, many older adults remain undernourished particularly those residing within a variety of institutions. Blechman and Gelb (1999) identified that 50% of older people in institutions had protein energy malnutrition, whilst 3% of non-institutionalised adults had protein energy malnutrition. Protein under-nutrition has been associated with an increased risk of skin breakdown and infection in older patients (Wells and Dumbrell, 2006). In older adults, diseases tend not to present as we might expect (Wells and Dumbrell, 2006), for example ageing changes may be confused with signs of under-nutrition such as dry skin and loss of turgor. This adds to the difficulty in detecting and diagnosing patients who are undernourished.

Many factors are linked to the cause of malnutrition in the older adult (Wells and Dumbrell, 2006) whether they are in the community or in hospital. We refer you to the following list for a summary of such factors:

- Alcohol
- Drug misuse
- Medical problems, for example cardiac failure, stroke
- Dementia
- Social isolation
- Depression and other psychiatric disorders
- Poverty
- Food attitudes
- Cultural preferences
- Dental problems

- Poor vision
- Medication side effects
- Functional dependencies, for example dependence on others for activities of living
- Environmental factors
- Limited access to or intake of food
- Elder abuse
- Loss of carer
- The inability to no longer be able to drive a motor vehicle.

However, there are specific factors associated with being in hospital settings that add to the risk of older patients remaining undernourished whilst hospitalised. These include:

- Nausea
- Vomiting
- Nil by mouth orders
- The placement of food out of reach
- Limited access to snacks
- Ethnic or religious food preferences all of which can contribute to low nutritional intake whilst in hospital.

Malnutrition during hospitalisation is associated with increased length of stay, readmission, mortality, skin breakdown and infection (Wells and Dumbrell, 2006). Screening and assessment therefore are not once only activities, but should be completed on an ongoing basis. Screening and assessment should include a diet history that considers the following factors: number of meals, snacks per day, chewing or swallowing difficulties, GI problems or symptoms that affect eating, oral health and denture use, history of diseases or surgery, activity level, use of medications, appetite, assistance with meals and meal preparation, food preferences, allergies and aversions (Lueckenotte, 2000). Food recall may also be useful but this depends on memory and it may be difficult for people to remember what they have eaten and the portion sizes if it is not recorded timeously.

Anthropometrics (BMI, radius to ulna length and mid-arm circumference are measured) and laboratory results should also form part of the screening and assessment, these could include serum albumin and transferrin levels (Lueckenotte, 2000). However, despite being widely used, the serum albumin and transferrin levels are not particularly good indicators of early undernourishment.

Once a problem has been identified, there are a number of interventions that can be implemented to ensure older adults are receiving adequate amounts of food. Holmes (2008) suggests a number of interventions to encourage older people to eat (Table 6.8).

Food guide pyramid

The food guide pyramid illustrates the relative proportions of different foods that make up a nutritious, well-balanced diet. An example of the food guide pyramid is shown in Figure 6.2. An alternative pyramid specifically for older adults can be found at: http://nutrition.tufts.edu/docs/pdf/releases/ModifiedMyPyramid.pdf.

Table 6.8   Interventions to encourage patients to eat. (Adapted from Holmes, 2008.)

Sit at the patient's eye level and make eye contact during feeding
Mealtimes should not be interrupted
Encourage family members to visit at mealtimes
Identify patient's preferences for food and drink
Staff meal breaks should not be arranged around patients' meal times
Ensure good oral hygiene prior to and after meals
Remove bedpans, urinals and vomit bowls from area before meals
Improve quality provision
Ensure that cutlery and plates are clean
Offer nutrient dense snacks
Improve food service
Help those patients that require help to eat
Consider their sitting position, consider ability to manipulate food on plate, how to get the food from plate to mouth
If chewing problems are present a smooth moist diet may be helpful
Monitor hydration and nutritional status of dysphagic patients and liaise with speech and language therapist
Offer nutritional supplements
Provide small portions more often

Patients are advised to select the recommended number of daily servings from each of the five major food groups. If all foods from a particular group is not chosen, guidance should be sought in relation to ensuring all the nutrients required are gained. The recommended number of servings depends upon a patient's calorific requirements.

Constipation

The word constipation comes from the Latin word 'constipare' meaning to crowd together. Constipation can be described as infrequent, incomplete and often difficult passing of hard faeces. It can be uncomfortable and embarrassing for the person who is constipated (Holman et al., 2008). However, there can be liquid faeces if the patient has overflow constipation (Annells and Koch, 2002).

Constipation has not been taken seriously by health professionals despite it causing a lot of discomfort for the person who is constipated. It is not always considered of clinical importance which is why some older people use over-the-counter medications to self-medicate without consulting health professionals for help or advice (Ginsberg et al., 2007). Approximately one-third of affected individuals consult a GP for treatment of constipation (Pare et al., 2001). However, it is widespread in older adults' hospitals and care homes where 60–80% of residents are affected by constipation. This is compared to

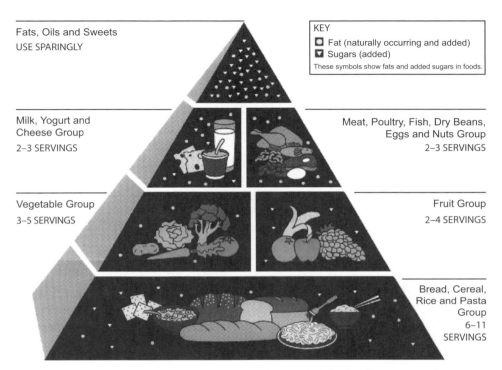

Fats, Oils and Sweets
USE SPARINGLY

KEY
☐ Fat (naturally occurring and added)
▼ Sugars (added)
These symbols show fats and added sugars in foods.

Milk, Yogurt and
Cheese Group
2–3 SERVINGS

Meat, Poultry, Fish, Dry Beans,
Eggs and Nuts Group
2–3 SERVINGS

Vegetable Group
3–5 SERVINGS

Fruit Group
2–4 SERVINGS

Bread, Cereal,
Rice and Pasta
Group
6–11
SERVINGS

Figure 6.2   The food guide pyramid. (This image is a work of the US Department of Agriculture employee, taken or made during the course of the person's official duties. As a work of the US federal government, the image is in the public domain.)

25–40% of people residing in day hospitals or living at home who are affected by this condition (Pare et al., 2001). Constipation is not only uncomfortable and embarrassing, it can be costly psychologically for the patient and also costly in the form of payments for treatment (Ginsberg et al., 2007). Constipation can also impact negatively on the quality of life for older people (Annells and Koch, 2002). An important issue that needs to be considered is the meaning of constipation to an older person in that they are very much individual to the patients and may not fit with the nurse's definition of constipation (Annells and Koch, 2002). However, some older people may have misconceptions that bowels need to open every day. Bowel movements range from three movements per day to three movements per week.

Constipation can be classified according to the categories seen in Table 6.9 (Ginsberg et al., 2007).

The diagnosis of chronic constipation depends on the persistence of at least two symptoms lasting for at least 12 weeks in a preceding 52-week period (Table 6.10).

Physiologically, defaecation begins when faecal matter moves from the small intestine to the large intestine. Peristalsis is described as a series of muscle contractions that propels faecal matter through the colon. Fluid is absorbed back into the body from the colon so that faeces are finally formed. Faeces are then moved into the rectum where a sensation

Table 6.9   Classification of constipation. (Reproduced from Ginsberg et al. (2007). With permission from John Wiley & Sons.)

Description	Definition
Severity	
Mild	>1 bowel movement per week
Severe	<1 bowel movement per week
Duration	
Acute	Constipation lasting < 3 months
Chronic	Constipation lasting > 3 months
Primary (idiopathic or functional)	Resulting from colon dysfunction
Secondary	Resulting from causes other than bowel dysfunction, for example physical obstruction of the GI tract, adverse effects of drugs and fluid restriction
Causes	
Slow transit	Constipation resulting from dysfunction of local intrinsic reflex mechanisms in the colon
Pelvic floor hypertonicity	Constipation resulting from hypertonicity of the anal sphincter and muscles used for stool evacuation

Table 6.10   Diagnostic criteria for chronic constipation. (Adapted from Thompson et al., 1999.)

At least 12 weeks, which need not be consecutive, in the preceding 12 months if two or more of the following symptoms are found in an adult: • <3 bowel movements per week • Straining during >25% of defaecations • Lumpy or hard stools in >25% of defaecations • Sensation of anorectal obstruction or blockade in >25% of defaecations • Manual manoeuvres to facilitate >25% of defaecations • Loose stools not present, and there are insufficient criteria for irritable bowel syndrome

of wanting to evacuate the bowel is experienced. The anal sphincter is a voluntary muscle that allows us to hold faeces until we can evacuate the bowel at an appropriate place and time. There is evidence to suggest that constipation increases with age, yet there are no physiological changes in the lower bowel to account for the increase in both self-reported and true clinical constipation among older people (McLane and McShane, 2001).

Causes of constipation in older people include colon disease, metabolic disturbances, neurological disorders, pharmacotherapy, inappropriate diet and/or fluid intake. Older people may voluntarily restrict fluid intake in the hope of reducing urological symptoms (Ginsberg et al., 2007), this in turn reduces the fluid content of faeces which contributes to the development of constipation. Polypharmacy may also be a contributing factor in constipation (Annells and Koch, 2002).

There are a number of causes of constipation such as mechanical obstructions, medical co-morbidities, medications and lifestyle issues. Mechanical obstructions include neoplasms or benign strictures related to diverticular disease. Medical co-morbidities will include stroke and PD. Medications are a major cause of constipation and older people are commonly prescribed three or more medications which therefore mean they are at risk of polypharmacy. Sixty per cent of medications including laxatives list constipation as an adverse effect. Most drugs that cause constipation interfere directly or indirectly with the physiological regulation of intestinal or colonic transit. Examples of medications with this effect include opiate analgesics and antimuscarinics. Other groups of medications that can result in constipation include anticholinergics, antidepressants, anxiolytics, antipsychotics and anti-hypertensives (Ginsberg et al., 2007). Lifestyle factors include limitations in mobility. Older people who rely on someone to help them to the bathroom may try delay evacuating their bowel which promotes constipation. Older adults may refuse oral fluids if they are at risk of urinary incontinence believing that this will limit their visits to the bathroom. Dehydration will result in constipation. The availability and ingestion of foods rich in fibre also needs to be considered.

Assessment

Assessment should include:

- Being asked to describe usual bowel habit. This should include how frequently their bowels open, use of any stimulants such as laxatives, any routines or rituals (e.g. reading while at the toilet).
- Find out changes in bowel pattern and record frequency and amount of faeces passed.
- Any pain on passing faeces?
- Any blood or mucus present?
- History and physical examination.
- History of bowel symptoms.
- Drug history including over-the-counter medications.
- Blood tests to exclude organic causes.

(Holman et al., 2008)

Kyle (2006) has developed a detailed risk assessment scale for constipation and are in the process of testing this tool for reliability and validity. This tool may be of use in the prediction of risk of developing constipation.

Management

It is important that health professionals acknowledge that older people have lifelong experience in managing their own bowel function and their preferences. Written information about constipation should be clear and understandable. It should be written in such a way that there are achievable solutions available. Health professionals should also be empathetic and understanding of the problems that older people may have regarding constipation.

The following advice should be given regarding the prevention of constipation:

- The importance of drinking 1.5–2 l of fluid every day
- Regular exercise within any mobility limitations
- High fibre diet including roughage from leafy vegetables, fruit and cereals
- Varied diet
- Be mindful of how often bowels open.

(Ginsberg et al., 2007)

Some older people depend on routines and rituals for the prevention of constipation, and these rituals should not be discouraged if they are safe and if they work. Breakfast is usually the meal that triggers the bowel reflexes and produces mass movement of faeces, forcing faecal matter into the rectum. Some individuals respond to a cup of coffee or hot water and lemon before breakfast.

Advice can also be given about positioning while on the toilet. Placing the knees higher than the hips in a squat position raises abdominal pressure and helps move the faecal mass into the rectum (McLane and McShane, 2001). If older people are taking opiates and have problems with constipation, then they should be advised to take a stimulant laxative with each opiate dose to prevent constipation.

Laxatives

Laxatives are the most common treatment for constipation used by participants. Older people purchase laxatives more often at a pharmacy than anywhere else (Annells and Koch, 2002). There are several different groups of laxatives including:

- Bulking agents (methylcellulose)
- Faecal softeners (liquid paraffin)
- Stimulant laxatives (bisacodyl)
- Osmotic laxatives (lactulose).

(Lueckenotte, 2000)

However, excess use of stimulant laxatives can lead to cessation of colon movement and the overuse of laxatives can result in constipation (Kacmaz and Kasikci, 2007).

Summary

For humans, eating and drinking is about more than just survival. Eating and drinking have a central role in many of our social and cultural activities. From an early age we learn that food and drink can bring us great pleasure. As we age, physiological changes occur that can affect our activity of eating and drinking. Many older adults do not consume an appropriate diet, often for a wide variety of reasons. Nevertheless, a balanced diet is essential to a healthy old age.

It is imperative that health-care professionals are familiar with and can select and use appropriate nutritional assessment tools. Good assessment skills are fundamental to assisting the older adults to eat well. If they are to eat well and to enjoy what they eat, a healthy mouth is imperative. Teeth, gums and tongue need to be healthy and for this reason we have given over a good sized section of this chapter to assessing and providing oral hygiene.

Many older people complain of constipation. Constipation is more common in older adults for a number of reasons. Health-care professionals must be able to advise on prevention and management of this potentially disabling condition.

References and further reading

Adams, R. 1996. Qualified nurses lack adequate knowledge related to oral health, resulting in inadequate oral care of patients on medical wards. Journal of Advanced Nursing 24(3), 552–560.

Annells, M. and Koch, T. 2002. Older people seeking solutions to constipation: the laxative mire. Journal of Clinical Nursing 11, 603–612.

BAPEN. 2003. The MUST Explanatory Booklet. Redditch, BAPEN.

Blechman, M.B. and Gelb, A.M. 1999. Aging and gastrointestinal physiology. Gastroenterology 15, 429–438.

Bowling, T. (Ed). 2004. Nutrition Support for Adults and Children. Radcliffe Medical Press, Oxon, UK.

Bowsher, J., Boyle, S. and Griffiths, J. 1999. Oral care. Nursing Standard 13(37), 31.

British Society for Disability for Oral Health. 2000. Guidelines for Oral Health Care for Long Stay Patients and Residents. BSDH, Newcastle.

Brown, B., Heeg, A., Turek, J. and O'Sullivan Maillet, J. 2006. Comparison of an institutional nutrition screen with 4 validated nutrition screening tools. Topics in Clinical Nutrition 21(2), 122–138.

Brownie, S. 2006. Why are elderly individuals at risk of nutritional deficiency? International Journal of Nursing Practice 12, 110–118.

Christiansen, J. and Grzybowski, J. 1999. Biology of Aging. An Introduction to the Biomedical Aspects of Aging. McGraw-Hill, New York, NY.

Clarke, G. 1993. Mouth care and the hospitalised patient. British Journal of Nursing 2(4), 225–227.

Curzio, J. and MacCowan, M. 2000. Getting research into practice: developing oral hygiene standards. British Journal of Nursing 9(7), 434–438.

Deems, D.A., Doty, R.L., Settle, R.G., et al. 1991. Smell and taste disorders: a study of 750 patients from the University of Pennsylvania Taste and Smell Center. Archives of Otolaryngology 117(5), 519–528.

Endacott, R., Jevon, P. and Cooper, S. 2009. Clinical Nursing Skills: Core and Advanced. Oxford University Press, Oxford.

Ginsberg, D.A., Wallace, J., Phillips, S.F. and Josephson, K.L. 2007. Evaluating and managing constipation in the elderly. Urological Nursing 27(3), 191–200.

Green, S.M. and Watson, R. 2005. Nutritional screening and assessment tools for use by nurses: literature review. Journal of Advanced Nursing 50(1), 69–83.

Harris, D. and Haboubi, N. 2005. Malnutrition screening in the elderly population. Journal of the Royal Society of Medicine 98(9), 411–414.

Heath, H. and Schofield, I. 1999. Health Ageing: Nursing Older People. Mosby, London.

Holman, C., Roberts, S. and Nicol, M. 2008. Preventing and treating constipation in later life. Nursing Older People 20(5), 22–24.

Holmes, S. 1996. Nursing management of oral care in older patients. Nursing Times 92(9), 37–39.

Holmes, S. 2008. Nutrition and eating difficulties in hospitalised older adults. Nursing Standard 22(26), 47–57.

Jones, C. 1998. The importance of oral hygiene in nutritional support. British Journal of Nursing 7, 74–83.

Kacmaz, Z. and Kasikci, M. 2007. Effectiveness of bran supplement in older orthopaedic patients with constipation. Journal of Clinical Nursing 16, 928–936.

Kenney, W.L. and Chiu, P. 2001. Influence of age on thirst and fluid intake. Medicine and Science in Sports and Exercise 33(9), 1524–1532.

Kyle, G. 2006. Assessment and treatment of older patients with constipation. Nursing Standard 21(8), 41–46.

Lueckenotte, A. 2000. Gerontologic Nursing. 2nd ed. Mosby, St. Louis, MO.

Mack, G.W., Weseman, C.A., Langhans, G.W., Scherzer, H., Gillen, C.M. and Nadel, E.R. 1994. Body fluid balance in dehydrated healthy older men: thirst and renal osmoregulation. Journal of Applied Physiology 76(4), 1615–1623.

Matteson, M., McConnell, E. and Linton, A. 1997. Gerontological Nursing: Concepts and Practice. 2nd ed. WB Saunders Company, Philadelphia, PA.

McLane, A.N. and McShane, R.E. 2001. Constipation. In Maas, M.L., Buckwalter, K.C., Hardy, M.D., Tripp-Reimer, T., Titler, M.G. and Specht, J.P. (Eds). Nursing Care of Older Adults: Diagnosis, Outcomes and Interventions. Mosby, St. Louis, MO.

Meiner, S.E. and Lueckenotte, A.G. 2006. Gerontologic Nursing. 3rd ed. Mosby Elsevier, St. Louis, MO.

Nair, M. and Peate, I. (Eds). 2009. Fundamentals of Applied Pathophysiology: An Essential Guide for Nursing Students. Wiley-Blackwell, Chichester, p. 283, figure 11.12.

National Nursing Midwifery and Health Visiting Advisory Committee. 2002. Promoting Nutrition for Older Adult Inpatients in NHS Hospitals in Scotland. Scottish Executive, Edinburgh.

NHS Quality Improvement Scotland. 2003. Food Fluid and Nutritional Care. NHS Quality Improvement, Scotland.

NICE. 2006. Nutrition Support for Adults. Oral Nutrition Support, Enteral Feeding and Parenteral Nutrition. CG32 National Collaborating Centre for Acute Care, London.

Nicol, M., Bavin, C., Bedford-Turner, S., Cronin, P. and Rawlings-Anderson, K. 2000. Essential Nursing Skills. Mosby Harcourt, London, pp. 119–201.

Pare, P., Ferazzi, S., Thompson, W.G., Irvine, E.J. and Rance, L. 2001. An epidemiological survey of constipation in Canada: definitions, rates, demographics and predictors of health care seeking. American Journal of Gastroenterology 96(11), 3130–3137.

Rattenbury, N., Mooney, G. and Bowen, J. 1999. Oral assessment and care for inpatients. Nursing Times 95(49), 52–53.

Roach, S. 2001. Introductory Gerontological Nursing. Lippincott, Philadelphia, PA.

Roberts, J. 2000a. Developing an oral assessment and intervention tool for older people: 3. British Journal of Nursing 9(19), 2073–2078.

Roberts, J. 2000b. Developing an oral assessment and intervention tool for older people: 2. British Journal of Nursing 9(18), 2033–2040.

Seeley, R.R., Stephens, T.D. and Tate, P. 2003. Anatomy and Physiology. 6th ed. McGraw-Hill, Boston, MA.

Simons, D., Kidd, E. and Beighton, D. 1999. Oral health of elderly occupants in residential homes. Lancet 353(9166), 1761.

Thompson, W.G., Longstreth, G.F., Drossman, D.A., Heaton, K.W., Irvine, E.J. and Muller-Lissner, S.A. 1999. Functional bowel disorders and functional abdominal pain. Gut 45(Suppl. 2), II43–II47.

Thurgood, G. 1994. Nurse maintenance of oral hygiene. British Journal of Nursing 3(7), 332–353.

Timiras, P. 2003. The gastrointestinal tract and the liver. In Timiras, P. (Ed). Physiological Basis of Aging and Geriatrics. 3rd ed. CRC Press, Boca Raton, FL.

Tortora, G. 2005. Principals of Human Anatomy. 10th ed. Wiley, Hoboken, NJ.

Waugh, A. and Grant, A. 2006. Ross and Wilson Anatomy and Physiology in Health and Illness. Churchill Livingstone Elsevier, Edinburgh.

Wells, J.L. and Dumbrell, A.C. 2006. Nutrition and aging: assessment and treatment of compromised nutritional status in frail elderly patients. Clinical Interventions in Aging 1(1), 67–79.

White, R. 2000. Nurse assessment of oral health: a review of practice and education. British Journal of Nursing 9(5), 260–266.

Winkley, G., Brown, J. and Stone, T. 1993. Intervention to improve oral care: the nursing assistant's role. Journal of Gerontological Nursing 19, 47–48.

Xavier, G. 2000. The importance of mouth care in preventing infection. Nursing Standard 14(18), 47–51.

Useful websites

Age Concern: Eat Well Leaflet. http://www.ageconcern.org.uk/AgeConcern/Documents/Eat_well_age_well.pdf.

BAPEN: The Must Toolkit. http://www.bapen.org.uk/musttoolkit.html.

Chapter 7

Eliminating

Aims

After reading this chapter you will be able to discuss the structure and function of the urinary system and relate this to the activity of eliminating.

Learning Outcomes

After completion of this chapter you will be able to:

- Describe the normal structure and function of the urinary system
- Conduct a comprehensive patient assessment of the above system using appropriate tools
- Detail the changes in the above systems that are associated with ageing
- Discuss the presentation and management of some common health problems related to the above systems that occur in older adults.

Introduction

As the digestive system has been discussed earlier, refer to Chapter 6 for information regarding the elimination of waste products via the digestive system. In this chapter, we will focus on the elimination of waste via the urinary system and, therefore, we begin with an overview of the normal anatomy and physiology of the urinary system.

Urinary assessment tools will be described and analysed in relation to their use with older people.

We then describe the ageing changes throughout the renal system and discuss their effects on the older person's ability to produce, store and eliminate urine.

Common problems associated with micturition and older people will be identified. For example, this will include urinary continence and UTI. We will then go on to discuss the

---

The Physiological Effects of Ageing: Implications for Nursing Practice, First Edition
© Alistair Farley, Ella McLafferty and Charles Hendry
Published 2011 by Blackwell Publishing Ltd

renal support older patients require both in the community and in hospital settings. This chapter will conclude with an examination of the nursing interventions that are required for older adults to attain and maintain adequate renal function.

Normal structure and function of the urinary system

The urinary system is composed of two kidneys, two ureters, one urinary bladder and one urethra. Collectively, the renal system produces and excretes urine from the body, it is involved in the regulation and maintenance of blood volume and blood pressure, helps regulate blood pH and involved in the regulation of several ions within the body, namely sodium, potassium, chloride, phosphate and calcium. The urinary system also produces hormones including erythropoietin (necessary for blood cell production) and calcitrol (an active form of vitamin D).

Blood supply to the kidneys

The kidneys receive oxygenated blood through the renal arteries. They receive 25% of normal cardiac output every minute which accounts for 1200 ml of blood (Tortora and Grabowski, 2004). Deoxygenated blood leaves the kidneys via the renal veins which drain into the inferior vena cava.

The kidneys are ~11-cm long, 6-cm wide and 3-cm thick (Watson, 2005). Each kidney is embedded in peri-renal fat which acts as a cushion, thereby protecting the kidneys from external impact. Internally, the kidneys are divided into two regions – the renal cortex and the renal medulla. The cortex forms the outer region and the medulla forms the inner region of the kidneys. Within these two regions are the functional units of the kidney. These units are the microscopic structures called nephrons. Each kidney has ~1 million nephrons. These are the structures involved in the production of urine from blood and the return of water and solutes to the blood.

Nephrons are composed of two distinct parts (Figure 7.1) – the renal corpuscle which acts as a filter for blood, and the renal tubule which contains this newly filtered fluid which is now referred to as filtrate. This filtrate is neither blood nor urine but an 'in-between' fluid contained within the renal tubule. It is from this fluid that urine is finally formed. Within the renal tubule, dissolved substances and much water in the filtrate are re-absorbed back into blood and other dissolved substances are secreted from the blood in the surrounding blood capillaries into this filtrate. These processes are essential in order to maintain fluid and electrolyte balance and blood pH.

The renal corpuscle is composed of a glomerulus (a collection of blood capillaries) contained within a glomerular capsule. This capsule is a double-walled cup of epithelial cells surrounding the glomerulus. It is within these structures that the first stage in the formation of urine occurs. This process is known as glomerular filtration. The filtration process results from differences in pressure within the glomerulus. The blood vessel entering the glomerulus (afferent blood vessel) is wider in diameter than the blood vessel leaving (efferent blood vessel). As a result of this, there is a build up in pressure within the glomerulus. This pressure eventually pushes fluid and small particles contained within

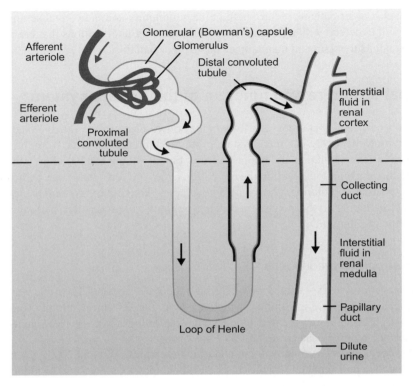

Figure 7.1   Diagram of nephron. (Reproduced from Nair and Peate (2009). With permission from John Wiley & Sons.)

the blood vessels to be forced through the walls of these blood vessels and the walls of the glomerular capsule in to the next part of the nephron. The fluid and small components forced into the proximal convoluted tubule (the next part of the nephron) are now referred to as filtrate.

The renal tubule is divided into three parts – the proximal convoluted tubule, the loop of Henle and the distal convoluted tubule. Within these parts, water and small components contained within the water are re-absorbed back into blood. In fact, 99% of water that helps to form the filtrate is re-absorbed within the renal tubule. In other words, for every 100 ml of filtrate that is formed, only 1 ml of that filtrate will become urine as 99 ml will be re-absorbed (see Box 7.1 for a list of filtrate components). Waste products not removed from blood through the process of glomerular filtration are removed by the process of secretion from the surrounding blood vessels (peri-tubular capillaries) into the renal tubule. Secretion is the opposite of re-absorption (Thibodeau and Patton, 2004), where dissolved substances move from blood into filtrate. These can include ammonia, hydrogen ions, potassium ions and certain drugs.

Distal convoluted tubules from several nephrons join to form a single collecting duct. Urine from the collecting duct now exits the renal pyramid into the calyx and renal pelvis before flowing into the ureter (for composition of urine see Box 7.2).

Box 7.1   Composition of glomerular filtrate

Glucose
Amino acids
Fatty acids
Salts (e.g. sodium and potassium)
Urea (from breakdown of proteins)
Uric acid (from breakdown of proteins)
Water

Box 7.2   Composition of urine

96% water
Salts – mainly sodium chloride
Waste products of protein breakdown:
   Urea
   Uric acid
   Creatinine
NB: Urine should not contain blood cells, protein, glucose or ketones.

The glomerular filtration rate (GFR) refers to the amount of filtrate that forms in both kidneys every minute. In males, this amount is ~125 ml per minute, and females produce ~105 ml per minute (Tortora and Grabowski, 2004). The GFR has to be constant. If the GFR is too high, the tubules do not get the necessary time to re-absorb substances and water, and as a result, these necessary substances and excess water are removed from the body. If the GFR falls, the speed at which fluid and its solutes pass through the renal tubules also decreases. As a consequence of this reduction, more time is allowed for re-absorption of dissolved substances and water. The result of which is that waste products are re-absorbed rather than excreted and more water is also re-absorbed, and hence less urine is produced.

Anti-diuretic hormone (ADH) is produced in the hypothalamus and stored in the posterior pituitary gland. ADH is released into the bloodstream when the water content of blood decreases even by a relatively small amount. It is also released in relation to a low blood volume. When it is released it has an effect on the renal tubules. It increases the rate at which water is re-absorbed. As a result of its release, more water is re-absorbed and hence less urine is produced. In the absence of ADH, less water is re-absorbed and hence more urine is produced and excreted from the body. This dilute urine will be of low specific gravity and generally colourless.

Aldosterone is a hormone released from the adrenal cortex. It is released in response to a low blood volume or a low plasma sodium level. When aldosterone is released, it also acts on the renal tubules enhancing the re-absorption of sodium and chloride with the added excretion of potassium. When more sodium is re-absorbed, more water is also re-absorbed. As a result of this, less sodium is excreted and less urine is produced and excreted.

Atrial natriuretic hormone (ANH) is produced by the atria of the heart. It has the opposite effect of aldosterone, where it stimulates the renal tubules to excrete sodium rather than re-absorb sodium. In this way, excess fluid can also be removed from the body.

The production and release of ADH, aldosterone and ANH are dependent upon body requirements and demands. When the body is dehydrated, ADH and aldosterone will be released (Tortora and Grabowski, 2004). On the other hand, if the body requires to lose fluid, ANH will be released and the release of ADH and aldosterone will be inhibited. ADH will also be released in response to raised blood osmotic pressure; a reduction in blood volume; pain or stress (Tortora, 2005).

Renin–angiotensin mechanism

When blood pressure falls, the kidneys respond to this stimulus by releasing the enzyme renin. Renin acts on the plasma protein angiotensinogen and converts it to angiotensin 1. This in turn is converted to angiotensin 2 by angiotensin 1 converting enzyme (ACE). Angiotensin 2 is a very powerful vasoconstrictor in its own right. It also stimulates the release of aldosterone from the adrenal cortex.

Aldosterone, as we have already seen, enhances the re-absorption of sodium and water from the renal tubules. This increased re-absorption of water adds to the volume of fluid circulating in the blood (CBV). In turn, the increased CBV increases venous return (the volume of blood returning to the heart), which increases stroke volume (the volume of blood ejected from either ventricle on each contraction). The increased stroke volume adds to the cardiac output ($CO = HR \times SV$) which in turn helps to increase blood pressure ($BP = CO \times PR$).

Activity

The renin–angiotensin mechanism is complicated and complex. In order to enhance your understanding of these processes, summarise the renin–angiotensin mechanism above into note form and list the events associated with this mechanism which will be initiated when blood pressure falls.

One ureter runs down from each renal pelvis on either side of the vertebral column and enters the urinary bladder. Urine is actively propelled down the ureters by peristaltic action, by the pressure of urine within these tubes and to a lesser degree by the action of gravity.

The bladder

The bladder acts as a temporary reservoir for urine. Its capacity to hold urine is between 700 and 800 ml (Tortora and Grabowski, 2004); however, we begin to experience the need to void when the volume of urine in the bladder lies between 200 and 400 ml. This initial experience of the need to void can be overruled if the time or place is not appropriate. This occurs because the external urethral sphincter muscle and muscles of the pelvic floor are under conscious control and the person can choose when and whether to relax these muscles. However, these preventative actions cannot last indefinitely and there comes a point when voiding cannot be delayed.

Three layers of the detrusor muscle (smooth muscle) make up the bladder wall. The lining of the bladder is wrinkled when the bladder is empty, lying in folds called rugae.

When the bladder fills with urine, these rugae flatten allowing the inner wall to become smooth. This action increases the capacity of the bladder to hold urine.

The urethra

This tube connects the bladder to the external environment. It is ~20-cm long in males and 4-cm long in females. The relative shortness of the urethra in females can contribute to an increased prevalence of UTI in women. The urethra has a single purpose in females – elimination, but a dual purpose in males – elimination and for the passage of semen.

Micturition

As the bladder gradually fills with urine, the pressure within it slowly increases and the bladder walls are stretched. When the volume of urine within the bladder reaches between 200 and 400 ml, stretch receptors within the bladder wall are stimulated. Sensory impulses are then sent to the sacral segment of the spinal cord.

This incoming sensory information is integrated within the sacral segment of the spinal cord. Sensory impulses are also sent to the cerebral cortex, which initiates a conscious desire to expel urine. Once the sensory information has been integrated within the sacral segment of the spinal cord, the micturition reflex is initiated.

Parasympathetic impulses are sent to muscles in the bladder wall and to the internal urethral sphincter. The muscles in the bladder wall contract and the internal urethral sphincter relaxes (autonomic reflex). The cerebral cortex now initiates, if desired, voluntary relaxation of the external urethral sphincter and urination takes place.

Ageing changes in the urinary system

The urinary tract is directly and indirectly affected by ageing. Direct effects are typified by intrinsic cellular changes involving nephrons and the muscles of the bladder. Indirect effects may be secondary to cardiovascular, endocrine or metabolic alterations associated with the ageing process (Timiras and Leary, 2003). The age of onset of change, the speed of change and the overall course of change and its consequences differ between individuals.

From the age of 30, renal function gradually decreases and by the age of 80 it is reduced by one half (Timiras and Leary, 2003). The decline in renal function is associated with a gradual loss of nephrons and a reduction in enzymatic and metabolic activity of cells of the renal tubules. This decrease in renal function can also be associated with pathophysiological changes such as atherosclerosis, resulting in a reduction in blood flow to the kidneys. Indeed, renal blood flow can be decreased significantly as the ageing process progresses. However, ageing kidneys continue to function normally (Christiansen and Grzybowski, 1999).

As previously stated, each kidney has at least 1,000,000 nephrons. As adults age, they can lose as much as 50% of these nephrons (Heath and Schofield, 1999); however, Christiansen and Grzybowski (1999) state that older adults normally lose about 25% of their nephrons. This loss normally has little impact on the body's ability to regulate body fluids. As a result, adequate fluid homeostasis is generally maintained in later life.

A decrease in kidney weight of 20–30% occurs, with the loss primarily occurring in the cortex. Also associated with the ageing process is a decrease of ~20% in kidney size (Christiansen and Grzybowski, 1999). With increasing age, the glomeruli and associated nephrons are replaced by scar tissue (5–37% between the ages of 40 and 90 years).

Glomerular filtration rate

Ageing results in a gradual reduction in renal blood flow, GFR, sodium excretion and re-absorptive ability of the renal tubules (Forrest, 2000; Muhlberg and Platt, 1999). The loss in numbers of functional nephrons reduces the GFR. Timiras and Leary (2003) state that the decrease in glomerular function may be primarily due to a loss or alteration of glomeruli and secondary alterations in blood flow. Glomerular filtration appears to be affected at an earlier age, and more severely, than tubular re-absorption and secretion. GFR and renal blood flow decrease progressively and significantly as one ages. Christiansen and Grzybowski (1999) state that GFR gradually decreases from the age of 30 until about 45 and that it continues to decrease more rapidly thereafter.

These changes result in a decrease in GFR after the age of 40, equivalent to 1% per year (Heath and Schofield, 1999). Furthermore, in the presence of decreased cardiac output (associated with changes within the cardiovascular system), the elimination of waste is also reduced. Creatinine clearance can be used as a measure of the effectiveness of GFR. Creatinine clearance declines from 140 ml/minute at the age of 29 to 97 ml/minute at the age of 80 in 30% of people (Christiansen and Grzybowski, 1999). However, these changes have little impact on the well-being of older people.

Changes associated with ageing in glomerular function do not pose any threat to well-being, likewise despite loss of nephrons and a reduction in GFR, renal function is not compromised by ageing. However, problems may occur when intrinsic renal disease exists or other factors such as inappropriate diet contribute to renal dysfunction. Diets high in protein may induce glomerular damage; conversely, a reduction in protein intake can reduce this damage (Timiras and Leary, 2003).

Creatinine

Creatinine is a breakdown product of skeletal muscle. Associated with the ageing process is a reduction in overall skeletal muscle mass. The reduction in the urinary output of creatinine may reflect the reduction in skeletal muscle that occurs with ageing.

Day/night changes in renal function

A circadian rhythm of urine production is usually established by 5 years of age (Ali and Snape, 2004). During adulthood, 75% or more of daily urine production and output occurs during the day, that is, 25% or less of urine production occurs during the night. Kidneys will concentrate urine produced overnight so that voiding is not necessary. After the age of 60, a change to more nocturnal urine production occurs. The ratio of day to night urine flow falls until the latter equals or exceeds the former. The kidneys also lose their ability to concentrate urine overnight and as a result the need to void increases. However, the total 24 hour urine excretion does not change (Ali and Snape, 2004).

This change in urine production and output has been associated with a decrease in renal-concentrating capacity, sodium-conserving ability and decreased secretion in the renin–angiotensin/aldosterone mechanism. A reduced action of the renin–angiotensin mechanism leads to a reduction in the amount of sodium re-absorbed within the renal tubules. This in turn reduces the volume of water re-absorbed within the tubules and, consequently, more urine is produced and excreted. The change in ratio of day to night urine produced and excreted may also involve the hormonal influence of ADH, where there may be a deficiency in its production and secretion (Ali and Snape, 2004; Timiras and Leary, 2003). A reduction of ADH secretion leads to less water being re-absorbed within the renal tubules and therefore an increase in urinary output.

As stated earlier, the ability to concentrate urine may be gradually lost, with the result that older people may be unable to cope optimally with dehydration or fluid overload. Provided the total water intake is 2.5–3 l daily, renal function will be adequate (Timiras and Leary, 2003). Problems may arise when water intake is reduced as a result of social isolation, reduced mobility, confusion, a reduction in the thirst mechanism associated with ageing or fear of incontinence (Timiras and Leary, 2003). In these instances, a reduced fluid intake will automatically lead to a reduction in GFR. This can lead to dehydration. This condition may also occur with the use of diuretics. Older people are also more likely to develop hyponatraemia and hypokalaemia during diuretic therapy as sodium and potassium are excreted in excess from the body.

Hormones

Christiansen and Grzybowski (1999) state that the distal convoluted tubule and collecting ducts probably lose some of their responsiveness to ADH, making it more difficult for water to be returned to the body, that is, more water is lost from the body. They go on to state that a decrease in sodium re-absorption across the loop of Henle can also occur. This can result in a reduction in the volume of fluid being re-absorbed into the body. As a consequence of this, the person may experience a lowering of blood volume and of blood pressure.

Several of the hormonal functions of the kidney have been shown to decline with age (Christiansen and Grzybowski, 1999). Renin secreted by the juxta-glomerular cells and aldosterone secreted from the adrenal glands both decrease with age. A reduction in renin and aldosterone will lead to an increase in urinary output and an increase in sodium excretion.

Anti-diuretic hormone is the main hormone responsible for the regulation of urine production (Ali and Snape, 2004). During the hours of sleep, there is a circadian rhythm of ADH with peak concentration occurring during the night. With ageing, there is a reduction in nocturnal ADH secretion, resulting in day and night levels of this hormone becoming very similar. This will contribute to the increased urinary output overnight.

Atrial natriuretic hormone (ANH), through its action on the kidney, results in excessive loss of sodium in urine and an increase in urinary output. ANH levels have been shown to increase with age which can also lead to an increased urinary output.

ANH has been shown to interact with the renin–angiotensin–aldosterone mechanism (Ali and Snape, 2004). High levels of ANH suppress renal secretion of the enzyme renin, which in turn reduces levels of angiotensin 2 and of aldosterone. As a consequence of this reduction in aldosterone, urine and sodium excretion is increased. ANH also opposes ADH action in the kidney and inhibits ADH release from the posterior pituitary gland (Ali and Snape, 2004). Therefore, ANH may contribute to age-related changes in urine excretion, that is, an increased loss of urine and sodium from the body.

With age, there is a decrease in the ability of the kidneys to concentrate urine (Ali and Snape, 2004). This decline in renal-concentrating ability is thought to be related to a change in renal tubular responsiveness to ADH (Ali and Snape, 2004).

With normal ageing, bladder capacity and bladder compliance decrease as do urinary flow rates and maximal urethral closure pressure. Frequency of detrusor contractions and the volume of urine retained within the bladder post voiding also increase with age (Rutchik and Resnick, 1998). These factors interfere with the bladder's ability to store urine successfully (Ali and Snape, 2004). As bladder muscles weaken, changes in the bladder storage capacity occur and incomplete emptying may ensue. Hormonal changes associated with ageing in females affect detrusor function and sphincter mechanisms, resulting in an increased likelihood of urinary leakage (Rutchik and Resnick, 1998).

Common problems of the urinary system

In the following section, we shall go on to consider two problems of the urinary system that are particularly evident in older adults. These are urinary incontinence and UTI.

Urinary incontinence

Urinary incontinence has been defined as the involuntary leakage of urine, and it is a common health problem among older people (Mauk, 2006). According to Wagg et al. (2008), it has been estimated to affect ~20% of people living in the community and a range of 30–60% of older people living in institutional care. SIGN 79 (2004) estimates that urinary incontinence rises with increasing age where up to 46% of women and 34% of men over 80 will have urinary incontinence. It is generally categorised as being either transient or established based on its onset and aetiology. Transient incontinence is resolved following treatment and has been associated with many causative factors such as infection, drugs, endocrine disorder, reduced mobility and faecal impaction (Table 7.1). Poor management of patients who have transient incontinence can also lead to the diagnosis of established incontinence. If factors associated with transient incontinence are identified and treated without success, the incontinence is then considered to be established (Mauk, 2006).

Wagg et al. (2008) state that incontinence continues to be under-reported despite the significant impact on quality of life and associated morbidity. Many older people who are incontinent cope in silence or do not present for care (Dingwall and McLafferty, 2006). They may not receive the necessary treatment for their condition (NHS Health Advisory Service, 1997; Wagg et al., 2008). This not only negatively impacts on the life of the individual but also on the lives of their carers.

People who are incontinent require proper assessment and management. The NSF for Older People (DH, 2001) stated that integrated continence services for older people should

Table 7.1 Common causes of transient incontinence.

Common cause	Rationale
Delirium/dementia	Impaired cognitive ability causes problems in recognising/responding to the need to void
Infection	UTI can cause urinary frequency and urgency
Psychological	Depression may result in loss of motivation to maintain continence status
Medications	Diuretics
Endocrine disease	Hyperglycaemia, hypoalbuminemia and diabetes insipidus are all associated with polyuria which increases the fluid load on the bladder which increases the risk for urge and stress incontinence
Reduced mobility	Interferes with the ability to reach a toilet in time resulting in urinary leakage
Faecal impaction	Over-distension of the rectum or anal canal can obstruct the bladder neck resulting in retention of urine, overflow and urge incontinence

be established by 2004. However, they did not allocate any resources to promote this objective. Wagg et al. (2008) published results from their audit on continence care which indicates that although older people are asked routinely about bladder problems, this did not guarantee an assessment of the problem, nor lead to appropriate interventions.

In older people, the cause and type of incontinence is often undiagnosed (Wagg et al., 2008). This can impinge on its management as without a known cause, evidence-based, effective treatment cannot be provided. Several authors suggest that management of incontinence in the older population is all too often reliant on conservative methods aimed at containment (Thuroff et al., 2006). This suggests an almost inevitability of incontinence in older adults. Indeed, Stoddart et al. (2001) state that incontinence in older people is often viewed as inevitable, irreversible and as a normal part of ageing. This approach to management denies the older person who is incontinent from the more proactive and curative measures which are utilised with considerable success in younger populations who are incontinent.

Classification of urinary incontinence

There are four different types of urinary incontinence, namely:

- Stress
- Overflow
- Urge
- Functional.

Stress incontinence is where there is an inability to hold urine as the bladder fills up. Urethral pressure is exceeded by pressure in the bladder (Doughty, 2000) and urine is forced from the bladder. This is often due to an incompetent urethral sphincter (sphincter weakness) and usually occurs during exertion, or following increased abdominal pressure, for example, when coughing or sneezing or even when laughing out loud. This can occur in either sex, but is most common in women due to their shorter urethra (Palmer, 1996) and the physical process of childbirth, where the base of the bladder may prolapse slightly through the muscle layer of the pelvic floor, thereby rendering the sphincter mechanism incompetent (Palmer, 1996).

Overflow incontinence is due to obstruction to the outflow of urine during micturition. Bladder outlet obstruction can be due to prostatic enlargement (hypertrophy, carcinoma and inflammation), bladder neck narrowing (contracture) or urethral obstruction (urethral stricture). The bladder over-distends due to increased resistance to the outflow of urine, but urine tends to 'spill out'. The person typically passes frequent small amounts of urine (Doughty, 2000). Symptoms include frequency, dysuria (pain on passing urine), poor urinary stream, urgency, hesitancy and pre- or post-urination dribble. There is incomplete emptying of the bladder leaving residual urine behind.

Occasionally, rather than involuntary urine leakage, the bladder is unable to expel its urine. This is described as urinary retention. Retention is usually due to complete bladder outflow obstruction, for example, due to prostatic enlargement in males, but can occur in post general anaesthesia due to smooth muscle inactivity.

Urge incontinence may be idiopathic (without a known cause), or secondary to conditions such as cystitis (inflammation of bladder and ureters), urethritis (inflammation of urethra), bladder stones or neoplasm. With this type of incontinence, the urge to pass urine becomes overwhelming and urine is passed before a toilet can be reached. Urge incontinence is caused by early contraction of the bladder which is due to premature sensory impulses being sent between the bladder and the brain. These premature impulses indicate that the bladder is full when it is in fact not and the bladder muscle starts to contract too early (this is also called detrusor instability). There is an ever present desire to void (pass urine), which if not satisfied could lead to incontinence. Typically, the person complains of discomfort, frequency, urgency and nocturia (excessive urination at night).

Functional incontinence refers to incontinence associated with factors external to the urinary tract. These can include cognitive impairment, physical disabilities and environmental barriers (Ouslander, 1994).

Urinary tract infection

Normally urine is sterile, containing water, salts, urea, uric acid and other waste products. Urine is normally free from bacteria, viruses and fungi. Infection occurs when microorganisms, often bacteria from the digestive tract, colonise the urethra and begin to multiply. The distal urethra is commonly colonised by vaginal and/or bowel flora (Baileff, 1999). The commonest cause of UTI is *E. coli*, which normally lives in the colon. This organism is responsible for an estimated 85–90% of all acute uncomplicated UTIs (Baileff, 1999).

Activity

Identify which other microorganisms are most likely to contribute to a UTI in older people. You may wish to use the following resource to help you: http://www.merck.com/pubs/mmanual_ha/sec3/ch56/ch56a.html.

In most cases, bacteria begin growing in the urethra resulting in a urethritis. From the urethra, bacteria can migrate into the bladder causing bladder infection (cystitis). If the infection is not promptly and adequately treated at this stage, bacteria can travel up the ureters to infect the kidneys (pyelonephritis).

The way the urinary system is structured helps to prevent infection. The angle at which the ureters enter the bladder normally prevents urine from back flowing towards the kidneys, and the flow of urine from the bladder helps wash bacteria out from the body. In men, the prostrate gland also produces secretions that slow bacterial growth. In both sexes, immune defences also prevent infection. Despite these barriers, infections still occur.

Urinary tract infections are more common in women than men. Approximately 70% of women will develop a UTI in their lifetime (SIGN 88, 2006). However, the incidence of UTI in men rises with age and may be linked to prostatism and subsequent incomplete bladder emptying. In women, the risk of UTI increases with age and sexual activity. The prevalence of asymptomatic bacteriuria increases with age. The fact that women have a shorter urethra accounts for the increase of UTIs among women compared to men (Baileff, 1999). The close proximity of the urethra to the anus in females may also contribute to the greater risk of infection and bacteriuria in women. Rates of UTI are high in post-menopausal women because of bladder or uterine prolapse, causing incomplete bladder emptying.

A common source of UTI is indwelling urinary catheters.

Activity

Identify and justify measures which can be taken to reduce the risk of UTI developing in an older patient who has recently been catheterised using an indwelling urinary catheter.

Not everyone with a UTI will have signs and symptoms, but most experience some obvious features.

If a person has a UTI, they often experience a frequent urge to pass urine and a painful, burning sensation in the area of the bladder or urethra during micturition. However, despite the urgency, often, only a small amount of urine may be passed. The person may feel tired, tremorous, washed out and experience back pain even when not passing urine. An uncomfortable pressure above the pubic bone may also be experienced and some men feel fullness in the rectum. Infected urine may look milky or cloudy with a reddish tinge if blood is present. Bloody urine is reported in as many as 10% of cases of UTI in otherwise healthy women.

Table 7.2 compares possible signs and symptoms of UTI in adults and older people.

It should be noted that whilst pyrexia and dysuria are typical signs of UTI in adults, these are experienced less often in the older age. Symptoms such as falls, confusion, new onset of urinary incontinence, lethargy, nocturia and anorexia may be the first signs of a UTI in an older person (Lueckenotte, 2000; Naish and Hallam, 2007).

Activity

What investigations can be undertaken to assist in the diagnosis of UTI?

Table 7.2   Signs and symptoms of UTI. (From Naish and Hallam (2007), reproduced with permission from the RCN.)

Signs and symptoms	Adults	Older people
Dysuria	Yes	Possible
Frequency	Yes	Yes
Urgency	Yes	Yes
Loin pain	Yes	Yes
Blood in urine	Yes	Yes
Pyrexia	Yes	Possible
Abdominal pain	Yes	Rarely
Offensive smelling urine	Yes	Yes
Cloudy urine	Yes	Yes

Nursing management of UTI should include interventions that focus on education for older people. This includes good personal hygiene after toileting such as wiping from front to back, a good fluid intake and reporting signs and symptoms of UTI.

Reflection Point

Consider the use of cranberry juice as a means of preventing or treating UTI. Identify the arguments for and against its popularity in the management of this condition.

 Point for Practice

Identify common drugs used to manage UTI and explain their actions.

Medications for the treatment of UTI are described in the SIGN Guidelines 88 (2006) and NICE Guideline 40 (2006).

Assessment of continence

Reflection Point

Consider how you currently assess your patient's levels of continence. Are any protocols and guidelines regarding urinary continence in older people available to assist you? Reflect upon the usefulness of such protocols and guidelines in directing care.

A number of incontinence assessment tools have been developed, many of which were devised for women but have since been adapted for men. Many of these tools have also been tested for reliability and validity. However, there appears to be no tool specifically designed for older people.

Assessment should include full history, pelvic floor assessment in both sexes, digital rectal examination for prostate size, shape and consistency, urine testing, midstream specimen of urine (MSU) for culture and sensitivity if required and voiding patterns (SIGN, 79, 2004).

Both NICE (2006) and SIGN (2004) recommend a number of different urinary continence assessment tools. These tools are widely available and generally easy to administer. Some of these tools will be described here, but we recommend readers to access the NICE and SIGN websites for a list of recommended assessment tools.

Assessment of continence is an essential precursor to the planning of appropriate nursing care for patients experiencing urinary symptoms. A specific assessment of the person's pattern of voiding, as well as observation and testing of a sample of their urine is required. This allows for a full assessment of the elimination problem and helps establish realistic nursing outcomes.

During an initial assessment, the following should be considered:

- What is the time interval between voiding?
- What is the volume of urine passed each time? This therefore requires to be measured.
- Is there any prior warning to voiding – if so, how much warning is there before the need to void?
- Any experience of pain on passing urine (dysuria)?
- What is the overall appearance of urine – is it cloudy, concentrated, dilute, any presence of blood?
- Does the urine have a distinctive smell?
- Does the person experience any difficulty in starting or stopping passing urine?
- Any episodes of urinary incontinence?

Other factors may influence a person's state of continence. The following should also be noted:

- Environmental factors such as ease of access to toilets, the number of toilets available for the number of people in the environment, stairs to climb before reaching the toilet.
- Physical factors such as medications currently prescribed, limited mobility, manual dexterity, bowel habits, ability to engage in self-care activities, sexual dysfunction, clothing worn (buttons, zips and layers of clothing) should also be considered.
- Mental status may affect continence, for example if confused, agitated or suffering from cognitive deficits.
- Emotions such as stress can affect levels of continence.

Reflection Point

Given your growing knowledge regarding incontinence and the factors which influence this, how would you manage your patient's environment to minimise the risk of urinary incontinence.

The urogenital distress inventory

The urogenital distress inventory (UDI) was developed by Shumaker et al. (1994). It was designed to assess how urinary incontinence affected quality of life for women. The original form of the UDI had 19 items to assess, but work by Uebersax et al. (1995) produced a six-item version of the UDI. This is now accepted and widely used to assess urinary incontinence in practice.

Long form of UDI

The UDI items ask the respondent 'Do you experience and if so how much are you bothered by' which is followed by a list of symptoms:

Item	Not at all	Slightly	Moderately	Greatly
Frequent urination?				
A strong feeling of urgency to empty your bladder?				
Urine leakage related to the feeling of urgency?				
Urine leakage related to physical activity, coughing or sneezing?				
General urine leakage not related to urgency or activity?				
Small amounts of urine leakage (drops)?				
Large amounts of urine leakage?				
Night-time urination?				
Bedwetting?				
Difficulty emptying your bladder?				
A feeling of incomplete bladder emptying?				
Lower abdominal pressure?				
Pain when urinating?				
Pain or discomfort in the lower abdominal or genital area?				
Heaviness or dullness in the pelvic area?				
A feeling of bulging or protrusion in the vaginal area?				
Bulging or protrusion you can see in the vaginal area?				
Pelvic discomfort when standing or physically exerting yourself?				
Having to push on the vaginal walls to have a bowel movement?				

Short form of UDI

The six questions have the same items as reported above and cover:

Item	Not at all	Slightly	Moderately	Greatly
Frequent urination				
Urine leakage related to the feeling of urgency				
Urine leakage related to physical activity, coughing or sneezing				
Small amounts of urine leakage (drops)				
Difficulty emptying your bladder				
Pain or discomfort in the lower abdominal or genital area				

The UDI has been further developed to take into account the male aspects of urinary incontinence (Robinson and Shea, 2002).

The King's Health Questionnaire is recommended by NICE (2006) and SIGN (2004) as a useful tool to use when assessing levels of continence. This questionnaire was developed by Kelleher et al. (1997) to measure the quality of life in women of all ages who had urinary incontinence. They set out to develop a measure that was condition-specific as opposed to using a generic quality of life questionnaire. They produced a 21-item questionnaire with an age range from 18 to 85, mean 51.4. The questionnaire includes perceptions of general health and the impact of incontinence. It also includes the domains of role, physical and social limitations; personal relationships; emotions and sleep; perception of the severity of incontinence is also measured. A copy of the King's Health Questionnaire can be found in NICE Guideline 40.

A bladder diary is a useful component of a basic evaluation of incontinence. This identifies the frequency, amount voided and the continence status for each void. In this way, information is gained in relation to the severity of incontinence. Precipitating events may be identified, patterns to voiding problems may also be detected and any irritative or associated symptoms can be noted (Wyman, 1994). Doughty (2000) suggests that a 3-day diary will provide enough information to classify frequency and number of incontinent episodes. Patients and/or carers can complete the diary. Below is an example of such a voiding diary.

Voiding diary

Directions: Please print this form and complete the information listed below for three (3) consecutive days.

Date	Time AM/PM	Volume Voided (oz)	Amount of Leakage (1, 2, 3 below)	Pad Change (Y,N)	Urge Present when Leaked (Y,N)	Degree of Urgency (see 1–10 below)	Fecal Spotting (Y,N)

Urgency Scale
(No Urgency) 0 1 2 3 4 5 6 7 8 9 10 (Maximum Urgency)

Estimated Amount of Leakage:
1 = Damp
2 = Wet Underwear or Pad
3 = Soaked Clothing or Emptied Bladder

CONFIDENTIAL
(Reproduced with permission from Neotonus, Inc., http://www.neocontrol.com/patients/resources/voiding_diary2.htm)

Management of urinary incontinence

Once a thorough general and focused assessment has been completed and the type of urinary incontinence has been identified, there are a number of strategies that can be implemented to manage urinary incontinence.

 Point for Practice

Please use a voiding diary on three patients with urinary incontinence and use this information to guide your management of their incontinence.

Scheduled voiding

This strategy can be used to treat adults with urge and functional incontinence. Intact cognition is not necessary when using scheduled voiding. A schedule is established after using a bladder diary or by using common voiding patterns, for example, before or after meals, last thing at night before going to bed or whatever is normal practice for the patient. Thus, a patient will be taken to the toilet on a regular basis whether it is 2 or 4 hourly. If incontinence persists, then the schedule needs to be altered to accommodate this.

Prompted voiding

This combines scheduled voiding with monitoring, prompting and praising. Prompted voiding can improve continence in long-term care settings by between 25% and 50% (Ouslander et al., 1995). Once again, this strategy can be used with patients who are cognitively intact or who have cognitive deficits. The aim of prompted voiding is to increase self-initiated voiding and to decrease the number of incontinent episodes. The patient must be able to actively participate by agreeing to go to the toilet when prompted. If prompted voiding is going to be used, there must be consistency from all members of staff. However, a patient should never be forced to go to the toilet or should be reprimanded for failing to go to the toilet (Lueckenotte, 2000).

Bladder training

The aim of this strategy is to try and increase the time between the urge to pass urine and the voiding of urine. Thus, it is a useful strategy for urge incontinence (Specht, 2005). A voiding schedule is implemented until episodes of urinary incontinence stop. Once continence is achieved, then the periods between voiding are increased by asking clients to postpone voiding until the scheduled time so that they are voiding by the clock rather than the urge to pass urine (Lueckenotte, 2000). Patients need to be cognitively aware to participate in this strategy.

Pelvic muscle exercises

This strategy can be implemented if the client has stress, urge or mixed incontinence. SIGN (2004) states that the evidence is inconclusive for urge incontinence; however, a combination of pelvic floor exercises and bladder retraining may be useful. The aim of these exercises is to strengthen the pelvic floor muscles. This can be successful in all age groups and may be useful to men who have undergone prostatectomy (SIGN, 2004; Specht, 2005). Patients are required to be cognitively intact and the exercises need to be carried out from 30 to 100 times daily (Specht, 2005).

 Point for Practice

Identify the range of exercises which are beneficial in strengthening the pelvic floor muscles and develop a simple leaflet, with diagrams, for your patients to follow.

Intermittent catheterisation

Intermittent catheterisation can be used by patients or their carers for patients with urinary retention related to a weak detrusor muscle or patients with a blockage of the urethra. It can also be used for patients who have reflex incontinence related to disorders such as spinal cord injury. Intermittent catheterisation reduces the risk of an overextended bladder, consequently reducing the risk of urinary infection (Maas and Specht, 2001). Patients and/or carers need to have manual dexterity to manage intermittent self-catheterisation. It is a clean procedure as opposed to a sterile procedure; however, the procedure may need to be carried out 2–3 hourly with the process being carried out about twice during the night.

There are numerous drugs that can be used to manage urinary incontinence. See NICE Guideline 40 and SIGN Guideline 88 for a further explanation. If urinary incontinence is intractable, there are many good containment devices available. Wagg et al. (2008) demonstrated that containment devices continue to be the most popular strategy in the management of urinary incontinence. However, all efforts should be aimed at reducing the incidence and prevalence of urinary incontinence, and containment devices should be seen as a last resort as opposed to the first-line management of urinary incontinence.

Activity

Identify common drugs used to manage urinary incontinence and explain their actions.

Fonda et al. (1998) identified that little work has been carried out on the prevention of urinary incontinence in older people. However, work done includes:

Primary prevention measures:

- Interventions that prevent predisposing conditions, for example,
  — Childbirth trauma
  — Pelvic muscle weakness
  — Detrusor over-activity
  — Impaired mobility
  — Staying mentally active.

Secondary prevention measures:

- Reversing the predisposing condition
- Preventing the progression to incontinence.

Tertiary prevention measures:

- Management strategies to decrease the severity and sequelae of incontinence, such as regular toileting programming and social continence using various aids.

Summary

The urinary system is responsible for eliminating waste products and excess water from the body. As our kidneys have a large reserve capacity, ageing does not normally carry with it any significant reduction in renal function. However, there are two conditions that, whilst not restricted to older adults, are particularly problematic in older people, namely incontinence and UTI.

Incontinence exists in a number of different forms and can be very disabling especially from a psychosocial perspective. Incontinence is not and must never be seen as a normal consequence of ageing. Older people should not feel that they have to accept this condition as part of 'growing old'. Health-care professionals should be familiar with the types and range of interventions and services that may be helpful in responding to this problem.

Urinary tract infection can also be very disabling. The typical clinical features of an infection of the urinary tract may not be evident in older adults. This condition may also predispose the older person to falling, another potentially life-threatening problem of ageing.

References and further reading

Ali, A. and Snape, J. 2004. Nocturia in older people: a review of causes, consequences, assessment and management. International Journal of Clinical Practice 58(4), 366–373.

Baileff, A. 1999. Identify and treat urinary tract infection. Practice Nurse 17(10), 689–690, 692.

Christiansen, J. and Grzybowski, J. 1999. Biology of Aging. An Introduction to the Biomedical Aspects of Aging. McGraw-Hill, New York, NY.

Department of Health. 2001. The National Service Framework for Older People. The Stationery Office, London.

Dingwall, L. and McLafferty, E. 2006. Do nurses promote urinary continence in hospitalized older people?: an exploratory study. Journal of Clinical Nursing 15(10), 1276–1286.

Doughty, D.B. 2000. Urinary and Fecal Incontinence: Nursing Management. 2nd ed. Mosby, St. Louis, MO.

Fonda, D., Resnick, N.M. and Kirschner-Hermanns, R. 1998. Prevention of urinary incontinence in older people. British Journal of Urology 82(Suppl. 1), 5–10.

Forrest, J. 2000. Gerontological alterations. In Urden, L.D. and Stacy, K.M. (Eds). Priorities in Critical Care Nursing. 3rd ed. Mosby, St. Louis, MO.

Heath, H. and Schofield, I. 1999. Healthy Ageing: Nursing Older People. Mosby, London.

Kelleher, C.J., Cardozo, L.D., Khullar, V. and Salvatore, S. 1997. A new questionnaire to assess the quality of life of urinary incontinent women. British Journal of Obstetrics and Gynaecology 104, 1374–1379.

Lueckenotte, A.G. 2000. Gerontologic Nursing. 2nd ed. Mosby, St. Louis, MO.

Maas, M.L. and Specht, J.P. 2001. Urinary incontinence: functional, iatrogenic, overflow, reflex, stress, total, and urge. In Maas, M.L., Buckwalter, K.C., Hardy, M.D., Tripp-Reimer, T., Titler, M.G. and Specht, J.P. (Eds). Nursing Care of Older Adults: Diagnoses, Outcomes and Interventions. Mosby, St. Louis, MO.

Mauk, K.L. 2006. Gerontological Nursing: Competencies for Care. Jones and Bartlett Publishers, Massachusetts.

Muhlberg, W. and Platt, D. 1999. Age-dependent changes of the kidneys: pharmacological implications. Gerontology 45, 243–253.

Nair, M. and Peate, I. (Eds). 2009. Fundamentals of Applied Pathophysiology: An Essential Guide for Nursing Students. Wiley-Blackwell, Chichester, p. 193, Figure 8.4.

Naish, W. and Hallam, M. 2007. Urinary tract infection: diagnosis and management for nurses. Nursing Standard 21(23), 50–57.

National Health Service Health Advisory Service. 1997. Services for the People Who Are Elderly. The Stationery Office, Norwich.

National Institute for Health and Clinical Excellence. 2006. Urinary Incontinence. The Management of Urinary Incontinence in Women. Guideline 40. NICE, London.

Ouslander, J. 1994. Incontinence. In Kane, R., Ouslander, J. and Abrass, I. (Eds). Essentials of Clinical Geriatrics. 3rd ed. McGraw-Hill, New York, NY.

Ouslander, J.G., Schnelle, J.F., Uman, G., et al. 1995. Predictors of successful prompted voiding among incontinent nursing home residents. The Journal of the American Medical Association 273(17), 1366–1370.

Palmer, M.H. 1996. Urinary Incontinence: Assessment and Promotion. Aspen Publishers, Gaithersburg, MD.

Robinson, J.P. and Shea, J.A. 2002. Development and testing of a measure of health-related quality of life for men with urinary incontinence. Journal of the American Geriatrics Society 50(5), 935–945.

Rutchik, S.D. and Resnick, M.I. 1998. The epidemiology of incontinence in the elderly. British Journal of Urology 82(Suppl. 1), 1–4.

Scottish Intercollegiate Guidelines Network. 2004. Management of Urinary Incontinence in Primary Care: Guideline 79. SIGN, Edinburgh.

Scottish Intercollegiate Guidelines Network. 2006. Management of Suspected Bacterial Urinary Tract Infection in Adults: Guideline 88. SIGN, Edinburgh.

Shumaker, S.A., Wyman, J.F., Uebersax, J.S., McClish, D. and Fantl, J.A. 1994. Health related quality of life measures for women with urinary incontinence: the incontinence impact questionnaire and the urogenital distress inventory. Quality of Life Research 3, 291–306.

Specht, J.K. 2005. 9 Myths of incontinence in older adults. American Journal of Nursing 105(6), 58–68.

Stoddart, H., Donovan, J., Whitley, E., Sharp, D. and Harvey, I. 2001. Urinary incontinence in older people in the community: a neglected problem? British Journal of General Practice 51, 548–554.

Thibodeau, G.A. and Patton, K.T. 2004. Structure and Function of the Body. 12th ed. Mosby, St. Louis, MO.

Thuroff, J., Abrams, P., Andersson, K.E., et al. 2006. Guidelines on Urinary Incontinence. European Association of Urology, The Netherlands.

Timiras, M. and Leary, J. 2003. The kidney, the lower tract, body fluids and the prostate. In Timiras, P. (Ed). Physiological Basis of Aging and Geriatrics. 3rd ed. CRC Press, Boca Raton, FL, pp. 337–358.

Tortora, G. 2005. Principals of Human Anatomy. 10th ed. Wiley, Hoboken, NJ.

Tortora, G.J. and Grabowski, S.R. 2004. Introduction to the Human Body: Essentials of Anatomy and Physiology. 6th ed. John Wiley & Sons, New Jersey.

Uebersax, J.S., Wyman, J.F., Shumaker, S.A., McClish, D.K. and Fantl, J.A. 1995. Short forms to assess life quality and symptom distress for urinary incontinence in women: the incontinence impact questionnaire and the urogenital distress inventory. Neurourology and Urodynamics 14, 131–139.

Wagg, A., Potter, J., Peel, P., Irwin, P., Lowe, D. and Pearson, M. 2008. National audit of continence. Care for older people: management of urinary incontinence. Age and Ageing 37, 39–44.
Watson, R. 2005. Anatomy and Physiology for Nurses. 12th ed. Elsevier, Edinburgh.
Wyman, J.F. 1994. Level 3: comprehensive assessment and management of urinary incontinence by continence nurse specialists. Nurse Practitioner Forum 5(3), 177–185.

Useful websites

Scottish Intercollegiate Guidelines Network. http://www.sign.ac.uk/.
NHS National Institute for Health and Clinical Excellence. http://www.nice.org.uk/.
NICE: Urinary Incontinence Guideline. http://guidance.nice.org.uk/CG40.

Chapter 8

Controlling Body Temperature

Aims

After reading this chapter you will be able to describe the mechanisms for regulating body temperature and relate these to the management of thermoregulatory disorders.

Learning Outcomes

After completion of this chapter you will be able to:

- Describe the normal components involved in the regulation of body temperature
- Conduct a comprehensive patient assessment of the above systems using appropriate tools
- Detail the changes in the above systems that are associated with ageing
- Discuss the presentation and management of some common health problems related to the above systems that occur in older adults.

Introduction

The body's cells function best when maintained in a stable environment. One aspect of this environment is temperature. Body temperature reflects the balance achieved between heat produced within the body and heat lost. Ideally, body temperature should be kept between 36.2°C and 37.6°C (Thibodeau and Patton, 2005).

Normal structure and function

A number of structures are involved in controlling body temperature including the skin and the liver. The hypothalamus in the brain is largely responsible for regulating body temperature.

The Physiological Effects of Ageing: Implications for Nursing Practice, First Edition
© Alistair Farley, Ella McLafferty and Charles Hendry
Published 2011 by Blackwell Publishing Ltd

Structure of the skin

Structurally, the skin is composed of two parts, the outer epidermis and the inner dermis.

The epidermis is organised in four or five cell layers. Where the exposure to friction is the greatest, such as the soles of the feet (and the palms of the hands), the epidermis has five layers. All other parts have four layers.

From the deepest layer to the most superficial:

The **stratum basale** is a single layer which is capable of continued cell division by mitosis. As these cells multiply, they push up towards the surface of the skin and become part of the next layers.

The **stratum spinosum** contains eight to ten rows of closely fitting cells.

The **stratum granulosum** is composed of three to five rows of flattened cells that are involved in keratin formation. Keratin is a waterproofing protein found in the top layers of the epidermis. The nuclei of the cells in the stratum granulosum are in various stages of degeneration and as the nuclei breakdown the cell is no longer able to carry out normal/essential metabolic reactions and they die.

The **stratum lucidum** is found only in the thick skin of the feet and hands. It is composed of several rows of clear, flat, dead cells.

Finally, the **stratum corneum** contains 25–30 rows of flat, dead cells completely filled with keratin (waterproofing protein). These cells are continually shed and replaced. The stratum corneum serves as an effective barrier against light and heat waves, bacteria and many chemicals.

It takes about 2 weeks for a basal cell (cell from the stratum basale) to be pushed up into the stratum corneum and another 2 weeks for the remains of that cell to slough off.

The maintenance of a healthy epidermis is dependent upon the following being synchronised:

- Continual cell division in the deeper layers with new cells being pushed to the surface (stratum corneum)
- Effective keratinisation of cells as they approach the surface
- Removal of dead cells from the surface (desquamation).

The dermis

The dermis is a thicker layer of connective tissue that underlies the epidermal layer. It is composed of collagen (the body's main building protein) and elastic fibres. Contained within the dermis are several important structures. These include blood and lymph vessels, nerves, sweat and sebaceous glands, hair roots and sensory receptors (nerve endings).

Gaining and losing heat

Heat can be gained and lost in a number of different ways (Table 8.1).

However, the balance between heat gain and heat lost can be affected by other factors, for example, environmental temperature, clothing, ingestion of hot or cold liquids/food and level of physical activity.

Table 8.1　Heat gain and loss.

Heat gain	Heat loss
Metabolism	Radiation
Physical activity	Conduction
	Convection
	Evaporation

Body temperature is monitored and regulated by temperature regulating centres in the hypothalamus. The hypothalamus is part of the brain known as the diencephalon which lies between the cerebrum and brainstem. The hypothalamus has several important functions which are identified in the chapter dealing with communication. However, one of these functions is to regulate body temperature. Information about core body temperature and the temperature on the surface of the body is conveyed to the hypothalamus by thermoreceptors. Peripheral sensory nerves sensitive to temperature convey this information to the hypothalamic thermostat. Additionally, the pre-optic area of the hypothalamus measures the temperature of the blood directly (core temperature) (Saladin, 2001).

The hypothalamus reacts to this information by initiating a number of responses. When temperature rises, the body responds by making attempts to bring the temperature back to within normal limits. These responses are examples of negative feedback systems, where the body's response is opposite to that of the stimulus. When the body is too hot, cooling is achieved by increasing the flow of blood to the skin where heat is then removed from the body by radiation. Sweat glands are also stimulated and the release of sweat from these glands aids in this cooling process by evaporation. Heat is also lost through the skin by the processes of conduction and convection (Tortora and Derrickson, 2006). Simple procedures such as removing outer layers of clothes will also aid in heat loss from the body and ingestion of cold drinks will also cool the body.

When the body's temperature begins to fall below normal limits, the thermoreceptors again relay this information back to the hypothalamus which responds by stimulating several body effectors which when activated work together to bring the body's temperature back to within normal limits. These responses include reducing heat loss from the skin by vasoconstriction which reduces the flow of warm blood from the core to the extremity. This helps maintain blood flow to the internal organs, thereby helping to protect core body temperature. Piloerection also occurs, where the hairs on the skin stand erect trapping air between them which is then warmed and acts as an insulator (Neno, 2005). Skeletal muscle tone increases and shivering generates much heat where body heat production can rise to about four times the normal rate in just a few minutes (Tortora and Derrickson, 2006). The hormones epinephrine, norepinephrine and thyroxine all increase cellular metabolism which helps to generate body heat (Cuddy, 2004).

Increasing the number of layers of clothes, wearing a hat and ingestion of warm liquids/ foods all help to prevent heat loss and maintain body temperature. Older adults are particularly prone to hypothermia as they respond slowly to changes in environmental temperature. This is due to a number of normal physiological changes associated with the ageing process. These include a decreased shivering response to cold, a decrease in metabolic rate, a slowing down of vasoconstriction typically associated with cold environmental temperatures and a reduction in the perception of cold (Brooker and Nicol, 2003). In order to reduce the risk of hypothermia in older adults, a number of fairly straightforward and simple measures can be taken. These are discussed later in this chapter.

Shivering is the rapid, involuntary contraction of skeletal muscle that produces shaking rather than purposeful, coordinated movement [this increases heat production up to 18 times that of normal resting level (Seeley et al., 2003)]. Shivering is stimulated when the hypothalamus detects a decrease in body temperature <35°C (Edwards, 1997). The aim of shivering is to achieve a return to normal body temperature. Non-shivering thermogenesis increases during periods of colder weather as a longer-term solution. This involves increased sympathetic stimulation and thyroid hormone release, both of which increase metabolic rate. This increase in metabolism brings about an increase in heat production (Saladin, 2001).

The liver produces a large amount of heat as a result of the vast amount of metabolic activity that occurs within this organ. Indeed, more than 60% of the energy released by the breakdown, or catabolism, of the food we eat is converted to heat rather than ATP (Thibodeau and Patton, 2005). This excess heat is then transported around the body by the cardiovascular system.

The effects of ageing on the ability to maintain body temperature

As the individual ages, the thermoregulatory mechanisms become less efficient. This makes it more difficult to detect and respond to temperature variations.

Epidermal changes with ageing

As we grow older, the skin becomes drier, rougher and less able to retain moisture. Age-related skin changes start at about the age of 30 and result in decreased protection and increased susceptibility to injury (Holtzclaw, 2001), slower healing, reduced barrier protection and delayed absorption of drugs and chemicals placed on the skin (Lueckenotte, 2000).

Damage to the skin can be seen through skin tears caused by the simplest measures such as the removal of plasters or dressings. A decrease in the levels of oestrogen and progesterone, associated with ageing, influence the process of drying and thinning of skin causing the skin to appear pale and translucent (Roach, 2001). Blisters can also form easily as we age due to these ageing changes. The skin becomes drier and rougher due to a reduction in the amount of moisture present in the stratum corneum (Timiras, 2003).

Increasing age is responsible for a reduction in the rate of turnover of cells in the epidermis (Holtzclaw, 2001). There are fewer basal cells being replaced and the basal cells themselves take longer to reach the stratum corneum for exfoliation. The turnover of cells decreases by about 50% between the third and seventh decades of life (Lueckenotte, 2000; Timiras, 2003) and results in the epidermis thinning with age (Roach, 2001). Thinning of the skin is also influenced by the flattening of the epidermal–dermal interface (Christiansen and Grzybowski, 1999). This area of contact between the epidermis and dermis decreases with age, resulting in easy separation of these layers and increasing fragility of the skin (Lueckenotte, 2000). Increasing amounts of moisture escapes from the skin due to the thinning of the epidermis (Lueckenotte, 2000). The skin becomes less flexible, elastic fibres lose some of their elasticity and collagen fibres become increasingly tangled. The number of fibroblasts, which are the cells responsible for the synthesis of protein and collagen, tends to decrease (Matteson et al., 1997). All these changes result in the dry and wrinkled skin appearance found in older people (Christiansen and Grzybowski, 1999).

Langerhans cells are found within the epidermis and have a role to play in the non-specific immune response of the skin. The number of Langerhans cells decrease with age. This reduction in cells decreases the overall effectiveness and responsiveness of the immune system.

Melanocytes, also found within the epidermis, produce melanin which is the pigment that gives colour to the skin. The number of melanocytes reduces with age by ∼8–20% per decade after the age of 30, both in exposed and unexposed areas (Timiras, 2003). This results in a decline of as much as 80% of melanocytes between the ages of 27 and 65 (Christiansen and Grzybowski, 1999). The decrease in numbers in turn decrease the amount of melanin produced in the skin. This contributes to the skin becoming much paler in colour in an older adult (Roach, 2001). Although there is an overall reduction in melanocytes, some of the remaining melanocytes increase in size (Matteson et al., 1997). These larger melanocytes lead to uneven production of pigmentation so that age spots called lentigo senilis form in areas where these larger melanocytes are found. These areas incorporate those most commonly exposed to sunlight including the dorsal portion of the hands, the face, arms and legs (Roach, 2001). The overall reduction in the number of melanocytes and the volume of melanin decrease the levels of protection offered by the skin in relation to harmful UVA and UVB sun rays (Lueckenotte, 2000). The reduction of melanin and its protective action and the reduced immune capacity of the skin combine to increase the risk of skin cancer in older adults.

Changes in the dermis

Associated with age, the dermis decreases in density, loses cells and has a reduction in the number of blood vessels within it. As with the epidermis, dermal collagen volume reduces with age. The total amount of collagen decreases by 1% per adulthood year. Collagen thickens, becomes less soluble and more resistant to digestion by the enzyme collagenase. This thickened collagen is less pliable with the effects of ageing and as such predisposes the dermis to tear-type injury. Elastic fibres within the dermis also lose extensibility and contractibility. A consequence of which is skin sagging and wrinkling.

Subcutaneous tissue loss also contributes to wrinkling. Wrinkling is particularly noticeable on the face as the skin here is constantly exposed to the atmosphere. Creases and lines particularly appear in areas of expression and use. Frown lines and crow's feet appear on the forehead and at the corners of eyes (Roach, 2001). Loss of padding associated with reduced subcutaneous tissue, especially in the extremities, makes the arms and legs appear thinner (Matteson et al., 1997). This loss of padding also contributes to a greater risk of hypothermia, skin shearing and blunt trauma injury. Decreased basal metabolic rate and a reduced ability to regulate blood flow also contribute to the risk of hypothermia (Christiansen and Grzybowski, 1999).

The flow of blood to the tissues decreases with age and the number of small blood vessels decreases (Timiras, 2003). There is a greater vascular fragility, leading to frequent appearance of bruising (Lueckenotte, 2000). Tissue and blood vessel repair is protracted, leading to an increased risk of decubitus ulcer (pressure sore) formation and delayed tissue repair.

Changes in dermal glands

Sweat glands reduce in number or functional efficiency in older people who as a consequence produce less sweat. This decrease in numbers or functional efficiency also interferes with thermoregulation with reduced evaporation of sweat.

The number of sebaceous glands remains constant with age (Timiras, 2003). However, the glands increase in size, but the production of sebum reduces with age. The diminished sweat and sebum production contribute to dry and rough skin in older adults (Roach, 2001). This dry skin may precipitate itching, resulting in scratching, which can lead to cracks and breaks in the skin (Holtzclaw, 2001).

Changes in nails

Rate of nail growth decreases with age and they become thicker and more prone to easily breaking due to brittleness. Most nail changes are due to a reduction in blood flow to the nail bed. Ageing nails can also show an increase in striations (nail grooves) which can cause splitting of the nail surface. This splitting leads to a break in the continuity of the nail, thereby increasing the risk of infection. Toenails can also become discoloured and grooved and may accumulate debris under the nail (Matteson et al., 1997).

Changes in hair

Hair greying occurs because of a progressive loss of melanocytes from hair bulbs. The more melanin produced, the darker the colour of the hair. A reduction in production of melanin is associated with ageing. By the age of 50, more than half the population have at least 50% of their body hair coloured grey, regardless of sex or original hair colour. In general, both men and women change from darker, thicker and more numerous hairs to lighter, thinner and less numerous hairs with ageing (Matteson et al., 1997). Heredity also plays an important role in greying of the hair (Timiras, 2003).

Hair follicles become less active with age and are not replaced as efficiently, causing hair to thin. Body hair loss occurs in a sequential fashion from the peripheral parts to the centre of the body. However, balding patterns in men develop from the centre of the scalp to the sides of the scalp.

The hairs in men grow longer around the eyebrows, ears and nose and they also become coarser. Frontal recession of the hairline occurs in 80% of older women and 100% of older men (Matteson et al., 1997).

 Point for Practice

Consider the above skin changes associated with the ageing process and identify how nursing strategies can be modified to care for the skin of older adults.

Conditions affecting thermoregulation in older adults

In the next section, we will examine two conditions that may affect older adults in relation to the regulation of body temperature, namely hypothermia and heat stroke.

Hypothermia

According to Mallet (2002), hypothermia is recorded on 300 death certificates in the United Kingdom annually. Those are cited diagnoses only so it is possible that this represents the tip of the iceberg only. There may be many deaths related to, but not directly attributed, hypothermia that are not registered. Hypothermia has been described by Linton and Matteson (1997) as one of the most important causes of death in older people in the United Kingdom. In a developed country, there should be very few deaths relating to hypothermia, but older people are a susceptible group as they may not always be able to pay to heat their homes. Older people who live in milder climates are also susceptible to hypothermia during the cooler months of the year (Mallet, 2002).

Hypothermia occurs when there is excessive heat loss from the body, when the body is unable to continue to respond to heat loss or when the temperature regulatory centre in the hypothalamus malfunctions (Ramont and Niedringhaus, 2004). Environmental conditions such as extremely windy and wet weather can greatly accelerate the onset of hypothermia (Rosdahl and Kowalski, 2003). A common cause of hypothermia in older adults is due to prolonged lying times after a fall. This reason for developing hypothermia is a combination of changes due to the ageing process, decreased levels of mobility and the ambient temperature. A rapid response to falls in older adults will therefore reduce this risk. The development of hypothermia is usually unintentional or accidental (Black and Hawks, 2005).

Hypothermia is defined as having a core temperature of less than 35°C. It can be further divided into mild, moderate and severe where mild is 32–35°C; moderate is 28–32°C; severe is less than 28°C. Hypothermia has also been divided into different types described as primary and secondary. Primary hypothermia has been described as exposure hypothermia where it has developed after an older adult has been exposed to low temperatures in the environment or they have been exposed to an immersion injury. Secondary hypothermia has been described as urban hypothermia and is common in patients who are ill or infirm and patients who abuse alcohol and/or drugs.

Kare and Shneiderman (2001) use a different method of classifying hypothermia. They classify hypothermia as accidental, inadvertent and intentional. Accidental hypothermia is similar to primary hypothermia and is described as exposure to cold environments without adequate clothing. In the United Kingdom, up to 10% of community-dwelling older adults have body temperatures close to hypothermic levels. Inadvertent and intentional hypothermia are associated with the care of hospitalised patients. Inadvertent is most commonly seen in surgical patients resulting from exposure to cool environments, whereas intentional hypothermia is the use of bringing patients' temperatures down to hypothermic levels for certain types of surgery.

Risk factors for hypothermia

For normal thermoregulation to occur, heat production needs to balance with the control of heat loss so that a constant core temperature is achieved (Mallet, 2002). There are a number of factors that interfere with this dynamic balance in old age including ageing changes, social influences, disease-related changes and medications (Table 8.2).

Older people are particularly susceptible to accidental hypothermia because thermoregulatory ability is progressively impaired with age. There is reduced ability to generate heat because of a decrease in lean body mass, impaired mobility, inadequate diet and reduced shivering in response to the cold. Older people are also susceptible to increased heat loss through a reduced ability to vasoconstrict appropriately. They may have abnormal adaptive responses, and may be prone to exposure to the cold through falls or illness (Mallet, 2002). Table 8.3 identifies the clinical features that a person suffering from hypothermia may present with.

With body temperature falling, metabolic rate decreases and brain metabolism slows down. Mental processes and respiration also decrease and bradycardia occurs. Bradycardia is often followed by cardiac irritability and a susceptibility to arrhythmia, including fatal arrhythmias. At this stage, the patient may slip into a coma and death can result due to respiratory arrest or arrhythmia.

Core circulatory blood volume increases due to peripheral vasoconstriction. The kidneys respond to increased circulatory volume by increasing urine output, known as a cold diuresis. Large volume urine will be pale and dilute with a lowered specific gravity.

Hyperglycaemia is common once body temperature falls to 30°C. Hypothermia inhibits insulin release from the beta cells in the pancreas and increases the cells' resistance to insulin. As a result, blood glucose is not readily transported in to the cells and blood glucose levels rise (Brooker and Nicol, 2003). Coagulopathy (a disorder of the blood where it fails to clot normally) develops with prolonged hypothermia.

Assessment

Assessment of temperature includes using a low-reading thermometer. There are a variety of thermometers available for use including the tympanic thermometer that measures the tympanic membrane (at the end of the ear canal) temperature, and this is regarded as measuring core temperature which is important in detecting hypothermia. Before using the tympanic thermometer, it is worth checking if one ear is better than the other for insertion of the tympanic thermometer. The ear that has recently been resting on a pillow should be avoided, and the ear where a hearing aid has been recently used should also be avoided. Both circumstances can cause a rise in the tympanic temperature. The ear should be checked for wax and an ear that is inflamed should be avoided (Woodrow, 2006). If possible, it is advisable to use the same site and method consistently when measuring the temperature (Mallet, 2002).

The environmental temperature should also be considered if it is cold, and the presence of any of the signs and symptoms of hypothermia should be observed and recorded. Other information that should form the assessment includes background or social factors that may predispose to hypothermia.

(Reproduced from McLafferty et al. (2009). With permission from the RCN.)

Prevention of hypothermia

Hypothermia is a largely preventable disorder in older people. Nurses have a very important role to play in the prevention and early detection of hypothermia as there are a number of simple measures that can be taken to prevent the development of this problem. Nurses

Table 8.2   Risk factors for hypothermia.

Risk factors	Examples
Ageing changes	• Decline in heat production with age
	• Loss of fat and subcutaneous tissue
	• Decreased shivering and vasoconstriction
	• Inability to feel the cold as intensely
	• Lack of motivation to seek warmth
Social influences	• Inadequate income
	• Social isolation
	• Inadequate housing
	• Physical ability to maintain heating appliances
	• Homelessness
	• Mental illness
	• Alcohol intake
Diseases	• Burns
	• Psoriasis
	• Desquamating skin conditions
	• Nutritional deficiency
	• Acidosis
	• Sepsis
	• Hypoglycaemia
	• Diabetic ketoacidosis
	• Hepatic failure
	• Adrenal insufficiency
	• Hypothyroidism
	• Spinal cord injury
	• Hypothalamic dysfunction secondary to stroke
	• Anoxia
	• Uraemia
	• Encephalopathy
	• Tumour or other lesions
Medication	• Phenothiazines
	• Benzodiazepines
	• Opiates
	• Alcohol
	• Barbiturates
	• Clonidine
	• Lithium

Table 8.3 Signs and symptoms of hypothermia. (Reproduced from Worfolk (1997). With permission from Elsevier.)

Degree of hypothermia	Signs and symptoms
Mild hypothermia, 32–35ºC	• Cold skin, pallor • May not complain of cold • Slurred speech • Intense shivering • Uncoordination, slow gait, may stumble and fall • Confusion, disorientation • Apathy or irritability • Increased blood pressure and heart rate
Moderate hypothermia, 28–32ºC	• Very cold skin, increasing pallor • Puffy face, generalised oedema • No complaints of cold • Speech difficult • Shivering stops, muscle rigidity develops • Slowed reflexes, poorly reactive pupils • Stupor, semi-comatose • Hypnoea • Bradycardia • Atrial and ventricular arrhythmias • Polyuria or oliguria • Dehydration, signs of shock
Severe hypothermia, below 28ºC	• Extremely cold skin, extreme pallor, blue blotches, cyanosis • Death like appearance • Muscle rigidity may become flaccid below 27ºC • Comatose, unresponsive to stimuli • Areflexia, pupils are fixed and dilated • Apnoea • No detectable pulse, ventricular fibrillation

also have an important role to play in the education of older people in relation to hypothermia. Nurses, first of all, need to be aware of the age-related changes that can influence an older person's ability to keep warm, and secondly, they need to incorporate this knowledge when giving advice.

Older people should be advised to avoid extreme cold. They should dress warmly in a layered fashion. Wearing lots of layers of clothes traps the body heat more effectively than one thick layer. The thermostat at home in the living area should be set between 65°F and 75°F or about 21°C. The DH (2007) advises that the temperature in the bedrooms should be kept above 18°C. If the bedroom is cold, then extra heat can be provided by using a hot water bottle or an electric blanket. The two items should not be used together. In very cold weather, staying warm in bed is a very important goal, so additional clothes including bed socks and even wearing a nightcap may be useful. If an older person is unable to afford to set thermostats at the appropriate level, help should be sought from agencies to supplement their pension. Nurses should be able to advise older people where they can seek help if they are unable to afford to keep warm.

Emergency numbers should be kept in a safe and readily available place. Emergency numbers include plumbing, heating engineers and the relevant NHS helplines. It is also important that neighbours and friends visit regularly to make sure an older person is coping especially in the cold weather (Kare and Shneiderman, 2001).

Other issues that need to be taken into account include the type of heating that is being used. Some forms of heating are much more economical than others. There are government schemes to help older people replace heating systems if the heating in their homes is less than adequate. It is worth checking that older people can work the heating system that is in place and that it is well maintained.

Help the Aged (2008) offers the following advice that can be passed on by nurses to their patients:

- Have regular hot meals and drinks. Food is very important in the provision of warmth, so regular hot meals and drinks will help ward off the cold (DH, 2007).
- Buy easy to prepare hot food with plenty of carbohydrates and vitamins.
- Move regularly whether it is walking around the house or outside. If outside, it is important that stout footwear is worn to reduce the risk of slips or falls.
- Do not sit for too long at a time. The DH (2007) recommends that people move about at least once every hour.
- Wear thick socks and tights.
- Wear a hat and gloves when going outside.
- Take a flask of hot drink to bed.

When visiting an older person at home, nurses should:

- Take a room thermometer on every home visit to check the environmental temperature.
- Contact social services if there is a concern about whether an older person is having a problem paying bills or because there is a concern about their mental state.
- Review the person's medication.
- Review the person's alcohol consumption.

The DH (2007) recommends that all older people who are eligible should have the influenza vaccination as a preventative measure. They also provide a document on keeping warm, which is updated regularly as does the Scottish Government. This document not only gives relevant advice in relation to keeping warm in Winter, it also provides telephone contact numbers in relation to help and services for older people. According to DH (2007), there are billions of pounds of benefits that are unclaimed each year, and patients should be encouraged to find out if they are entitled to any extra benefits. There are also winter fuel payments of £250 that are not means tested and are given to households where one or more adults are over the age of 60 and are entitled to this annual sum. The payment rises for people over the age of 80. There are also cold weather payments when the weather is exceptionally cold to older people who are eligible for this payment.

Activity

Using local and national resources, prepare a list of agencies that you may contact to request assistance for a client/patient at risk of hypothermia.

Acute management of hypothermia

The aim is to regain a normal oral temperature of 98.6°F or 37°C. (Thompson et al., 2002). Monitor the pulse, blood pressure and respiratory rate ½ hourly to hourly at the beginning of treatment, then 1–2 hourly until temperature reaches 35°C (Brooker and Nicol, 2003). Core temperature should be recorded using a tympanic or rectal thermometer (Elliot and Kiran, 2006), although the tympanic membrane temperature is becoming the preferred option for recording core temperature. The readings from the tympanic membrane are slightly higher than oral temperature readings (Ramont and Niedringhaus, 2004).

The first consideration should be airway management, therefore, ensure the airway is open (Farley and McLafferty, 2008). Oxygen can be administered to correct hypoxia, which if not rectified can lead to inadequate cerebral perfusion (Brooker and Nicol, 2003). Where possible, the oxygen should be warmed and humidified (Elliot and Kiran, 2006).

Fluid administration may be required to correct dehydration; therefore, intravenous access should be established. Fluids should be warmed before being administered. Insertion of an indwelling urinary catheter is advisable in order to closely monitor urinary output, as the person may be at risk of hypovolaemia.

Blood glucose levels should be measured immediately as hyperglycaemia is common once body temperature falls to 30°C. Hypothermia inhibits insulin release from the pancreas and also increases the cells' resistance to insulin. Therefore, blood glucose levels rise adding to the risk of hyperglycaemia (Brooker and Nicol, 2003).

A 12-lead ECG and continuous cardiac monitoring should be undertaken as bradycardia is common in hypothermia (Brooker and Nicol, 2003). A number of dysrhythmias may be seen in the hypothermic patients, as cold disrupts the conduction system of the heart (Nettina, 2006). It is therefore necessary to monitor the heart's electrical activity. Patients with hypothermia are also at risk of atrial and ventricular fibrillation (Black and Hawks, 2005; Cooper, 2006). If the person has severe hypothermia, they must be moved very carefully as sudden and violent movements can induce cardiac dysrhythmias or arrest (Nettina, 2006; Rosdahl and Kowalski, 2003).

(Reproduced from Farley and McLafferty (2008). With permission from the RCN.)

Re-warming techniques

During this acute phase of management, the patient must also be re-warmed. The actual way in which the person is to be re-warmed is dependent upon the degree of hypothermia (Nettina, 2006).

Passive re-warming

These measures will be of particular use for patients who have mild hypothermia.

Cold or wet clothes should be removed and replaced with warmed clothes and the person covered with pre-warmed blankets. If wet, the patient should be gently dried. If the patient's condition allows, warming drinks can be supplied to aid with increasing body temperature. Skin should be patted as opposed to being rubbed vigorously as rubbing can send cold blood from the extremities to the person's core, further reducing core temperature (Worfolk, 1997). Single-use, disposable laminate blankets can be used to reflect all radiant heat back towards the body (Brooker and Nicol, 2003; Elliot and Kiran, 2006; Neno, 2005) and as such are very effective in reducing heat loss and increasing body temperature.

Active re-warming

These measures are best used for patients with moderate to severe hypothermia.

If possible, the patient can be immersed in a warm bath at 40°C (Black and Hawks, 2005). Warm air blankets such as the Bair Hugger (Williams et al., 2005) can be used to bring body temperature back to within normal limits. These blankets allow warm air to be circulated around the patient's body, thereby wrapping them in a blanket of warm air. Heated pads or blankets can be used to raise body temperature (Holtzclaw, 2004), and radiant warmers are another option to bring body temperature back to within normal limits (Black and Hawks, 2005). The radiant warmers are positioned 70°cm above the patient (Williams et al., 2005) and direct heat towards them.

Active core re-warming

These measures can be used to reduce the length of time a patient's temperature is below 32°C, and the aim is to reduce the risk of cardiac arrest (Brooker and Nicol, 2003). Intravenous fluids can be warmed using a blood warmer prior to infusion (Black and Hawks, 2005). The temperature of such fluids should be between 42°C and 44°C (Elliot and Kiran, 2006). If oxygen is required, it should be heated and humidified (Rosdahl and Kowalski, 2003). Peritoneal and gastric lavage and extra-corporeal blood warming, such as haemodialysis or cardiopulmonary bypass (Spooner and Hassani, 2000), can all be used to re-warm the severely hypothermic patient.

Speed of re-warming

Re-warming methods should be appropriate to the level of hypothermia; therefore, prompt and effective individualised assessment is crucial. The speed of recovery for hypothermic patients depends on the length of time they have been exposed to the cold and their state of health at that time (Neno, 2005). The effects of raising the temperature can increase the patient's use of oxygen substantially. The aim therefore is to increase the temperature by no more than 1–2°C each hour (Brooker and Nicol, 2003). However, Neno (2005) states it is important not to warm the patient too rapidly, suggesting that re-warming in mild hypothermia should be between 0.3°C and 1.2°C hourly. However, if hypothermia is severe with cardiovascular instability, rapid re-warming of up to 3°C hourly may be necessary (Carson, 1999).

If body temperature is allowed to increase too quickly, the consequences may be beyond the body's ability to adapt in time. Oxygen consumption, myocardial demand and vasodilation all increase faster than the heart's ability to compensate, which can result in the death of the patient (Brooker and Nicol, 2003).

During the re-warming phase, a phenomenon known as afterdrop can occur. This is thought to be due to peripheral vasodilation and the release of cold peripheral blood into the internal organs which results in a drop in core body temperature (Elliot and Kiran, 2006). This further cooling can compromise cardiac function. When active core re-warming is discontinued, blood circulating to the peripheries is cooled and returns as cold blood to the core. This can reduce body temperature by as much as 2°C. As a consequence, when active core re-warming is stopped, it is important to continue with active and passive re-warming strategies.

Heat stroke

This is a severe, sometimes fatal condition that results from the person's inability to regulate body temperature properly. This failure of thermoregulation can be the result of a number of factors such as old age, disease or failure to cope with excessively high environmental temperatures (Thibodeau and Patton, 2007). This condition is characterised by a body temperature $\geq$41°C, tachycardia, headache and dry, hot skin. A temperature >41°C may lead to convulsions and a temperature $\geq$43°C will lead to death (Dougherty and Lister, 2008). It is imperative that the body is cooled immediately and fluid replacement therapy commenced.

When periods of hot weather are forecast, health and social care agencies should take steps to identify older adults at risk and put in place preventative measures. Advice should be given on how to keep cool. When overheating occurs, it is imperative that the body is cooled immediately and fluid replacement therapy commenced.

The DH in England has a heat wave plan that includes specific advice for vulnerable older adults. This can be found at: http://www.dh.gov.uk/en/Publicationsandstatistics/Publications/PublicationsPolicyAndGuidance/DH_099015.

NHS 24 in Scotland also has advice for the public on how to respond to heat exhaustion and heatstroke: http://nhs24.com/content/default.asp?page=s5_4&articleID=493.

Summary

Failure to adequately maintain thermal homeostasis can place the older person at grave risk of harm. In this chapter, we have reviewed the means and mechanisms of thermoregulation and have considered the problems of hypothermia and heatstroke.

Hypothermia has been reported to be one of the major causes of death in the older population in the United Kingdom. This statistic is perhaps made more horrifying when we consider that hypothermia in the elderly is largely preventable. It is important that health-care professionals can carry out a risk assessment for hypothermia and can advise on preventative measures. They may also need to be familiar with initial and subsequent strategies aimed at safe re-warming.

We also know that older people are at particular risk from heat-related illness and death. As a result of ageing, the body's thermoregulatory mechanisms are impaired and older adults may overheat especially during periods of hot weather.

References and further reading

Black, J.M. and Hawks, J.H. 2005. Medical-Surgical Nursing: Clinical Management for Positive Outcomes. 7th ed. Elsevier Saunders, St. Louis, MO.

Brooker, C. and Nicol, M. 2003. Nursing Adults: The Practice of Caring. Mosby, Edinburgh.

Carson, B. 1999. Successful resuscitation of a 44 year old man with hypothermia. Journal of Emergency Nursing 25(5), 356–360.

Christiansen, J. and Grzybowski, J. 1999. Biology of Aging. An Introduction to the Biomedical Aspects of Aging. McGraw-Hill, New York, NY.

Cooper, S. 2006. The effect of preoperative warming on patients' postoperative temperatures. Association of Operating Room Nurses Journal 83(5), 1074–1088.

Cuddy, M. 2004. The effects of drugs on thermoregulation. Advanced Practice in Acute Clinical Care 15(2), 238–253.

Department of Health. 2007. Keep Warm Keep Well: A Winter Guide 2007/2008. DH, London.

Dougherty, L. and Lister, S. (Eds). 2008. The Royal Marsden Hospital Manual of Clinical Nursing Procedures. 7th ed. Wiley-Blackwell, Oxford.

Edwards, S. 1997. Measuring temperature. Professional Nurse 13(2), 55–57.

Elliot, E. and Kiran, A. 2006. Accidental hypothermia. British Medical Journal 332(7543), 706–709.

Farley, A. and McLafferty, E. 2008. Nursing management of the patient with hypothermia. Nursing Standard 22(17), 43–46.

Help the Aged. 2008. Keep Out the Cold. Staying Warm this Winter. Help the Aged, London.

Holtzclaw, B.J. 2001. Risk for altered body temperature. In Maas, M.L., Buckwalter, K.C., Hardy, M.D., Tripp-Reimer, T., Titler, M.G. and Specht, J.P. (Eds). Nursing Care of Older Adults. Diagnosis, Outcomes and Interventions. Mosby, St. Louis, MO.

Holtzclaw, B. 2004. Shivering in acutely ill vulnerable populations. Advanced Practice in Acute Clinical Care 15(2), 267–279.

Kare, J. and Shneiderman, A. 2001. Hyperthermia and hypothermia in the older population. Topics in Emergency Medicine 23(3), 39–52.

Linton, A. and Matteson, M. 1997. Age-related changes in the neurological system. In Matteson, M., McConnell, E.S. and Linton, A.D. (Eds). Gerontological Nursing: Concepts and Practice. 2nd ed. WB Saunders Company, Philadelphia, PA.

Lueckenotte, A.G. 2000. Gerontologic Nursing. 2nd ed. Mosby, St. Louis, MO.

Mallet, M. 2002. Pathophysiology of accidental hypothermia. QJM: An International Medical Journal 95(12), 775–785.

Matteson, M.A., McConnell, E.S. and Linton, A.D. 1997. Gerontological Nursing: Concepts and Practice. 2nd ed. WB Saunders Company, Philadelphia, PA.

McLafferty, E., Farley, A. and Hendry, C. 2009. Prevention of hypothermia. Nursing Older People 21(4), 34–38.

Neno, R. 2005. Hypothermia: assessment, treatment and prevention. Nursing Standard 19(20), 47–55.

Nettina, S.M. 2006. Lippincott Manual of Nursing Practice. 8th ed. Lippincott Williams and Wilkins, Philadelphia, PA.

Ramont, R. and Niedringhaus, D.M. 2004. Fundamental Nursing Care. Pearson, New Jersey.

Roach, S. 2001. Introductory Gerontological Nursing. Lippincott, Philadelphia, PA.

Rosdahl, C.B. and Kowalski, M.T. 2003. Textbook of Basic Nursing. Lippincott Williams and Wilkins, Philadelphia, PA.

Saladin, K.S. 2001. Anatomy and Physiology: The Unity of Form and Function. 2nd ed. McGraw-Hill, Boston, MA.

Seeley, R.R., Stephens, T.D. and Tate, P. 2003. Anatomy and Physiology. 6th ed. McGraw-Hill, Boston, MA.

Spooner, K. and Hassani, A. 2000. Extracorporeal rewarming in a severely hypothermic patient using venovenous haemofiltration in the accident and emergency department. Emergency Medicine Journal 17(6), 422–424.

Thibodeau, G.A. and Patton, K.T. 2005. The Human Body in Health and Disease. 4th ed. Elsevier Mosby, St. Louis, MO.

Thibodeau, G.A. and Patton, K.T. 2007. Anatomy and Physiology. 6th ed. Mosby Elsevier, St. Louis, MO.

Thompson, J.M., McFarland, G.K., Hirsch, J.E. and Tucker, S.M. 2002. Mosby's Clinical Nursing. 5th Ed. Mosby, St. Louis, MO.

Timiras, M. 2003. The skin. In Timiras, P. (Ed). Physiological Basis of Aging and Geriatrics. 3rd ed. CRC Press, Boca Raton, FL.

Tortora, G.J. and Derrickson, B. 2006. Principles of Anatomy and Physiology. 11th ed. John Wiley & Sons, New Jersey.

Williams, A.B., Salmon, A., Graham, P., Payton, M.J. and Bradley, M. 2005. Rewarming of healthy volunteers after induced mild hypothermia: a healthy volunteer study. Emergency Medicine Journal 22(3), 182–184.

Woodrow, P. 2006. Taking tympanic temperature. Nursing Older People 18(1), 31–32.

Worfolk, J. 1997. Keep frail elders warm! The thermal instabilities of the old have not received sufficient attention in basic educational programmes. Geriatric Nursing 18(1), 7–11.

Useful websites

Help the Aged: Keep Out the Cold Leaflet. http://www.helptheaged.org.uk/NR/rdonlyres/CA45F296-3E60-47CD-8E6F-4DE27F62962F/0/keep_out_the_cold_adv.pdf.

District of Columbia Department of Health: Hypothermia. http://dchealth.dc.gov/doh/cwp/view,a,1370,q,602598,dohNav_GID,1787,dohNav,l33139l.asp.

NHS 24 Hypothermia. http://www.nhs24.com/content/default.asp?page=s5_4&articleID=466.

NHS Choices Hypothermia. http://www.nhs.uk/Conditions/Hypothermia/Pages/Introduction.aspx?url=Pages/What-is-it.aspx.

United States Environmental Protection Agency Extreme Heat Factsheet. http://www.epa.gov/aging/resources/factsheets/itdhpfehe/index.htm.

Chapter 9

Mobilising

Aims

After reading this chapter you will be able to describe the normal structure and function of the locomotor system and relate this to the activity of mobilising.

Learning Outcomes

After completion of this chapter you will be able to:

- Describe the normal components involved in the activity of mobilising
- Conduct a comprehensive patient assessment of the locomotor system using appropriate tools
- Detail the changes in the above system that are associated with ageing
- Discuss the presentation and management of some common health problems related to the above system that occur in older adults.

Introduction

We will begin this chapter with an overview of the normal anatomy and physiology of the locomotor system. In relation to assessment, we will focus on assessing the older person for osteoporosis and their fall risk. As in earlier chapters, we will examine in some detail the effects of ageing on the locomotor system and identify their potential impact on an older person's ability to mobilise safely.

We will then progress to consider examples of common problems associated with locomotion and older people, for example, gait changes and the ability to react quickly to the risk of tripping and falling. We shall discuss the support older patients require in relation to maintaining adequate levels of activity in the community and in hospital settings, and

The Physiological Effects of Ageing: Implications for Nursing Practice, First Edition
© Alistair Farley, Ella McLafferty and Charles Hendry
Published 2011 by Blackwell Publishing Ltd

examine the nursing interventions that are required for older adults to attain and maintain adequate levels of mobility.

Normal structure and function

The locomotor system

Skeletal tissue

Structurally, the skeleton is composed of two types of tissue – cartilage and bone. Bone is a rigid, non-elastic tissue. The structure of bone may be considered by studying the anatomy of a 'typical' long bone.

 Revision Point

Draw a 'typical' long bone and write short notes about the following parts: diaphysis; epiphysis; epiphyseal plate; periosteum; medullary canal; hyaline cartilage.

The skeleton has many different functions, including the support of soft tissue and protection of inner structures. It stores and releases several minerals, including calcium, sodium and phosphorus, and produces blood cells in red bone marrow. The skeleton also acts as a store for fats. It provides attachment to tendons and muscles and finally, bones act as levers when muscles contract and these levers then produce movement.

Types of bone

There are two types of bone – cancellous (spongy) and compact (dense). Cancellous bone makes up most of the tissue in short, flat and irregular bones and provide some support and a storage area for bone marrow. Compact bone offers protection and supports the body. Compact bone also helps the long bones, such as the femur, resist the stress of weight bearing.

Cancellous bone contains many spaces filled with red bone marrow (the cells of which are responsible for the production of blood cells). Compact bone is much denser and is made up from structures known as Haversian systems or osteons.

Blood vessels, lymphatic vessels and nerves from the periosteum penetrate compact bone through perforating canals. These vessels and nerves then connect with central (Haversian) canals running longitudinally through the bone. Surrounding these central canals are rings of hard calcified matrix called lamellae. Between the lamellae are spaces containing mature bone cells known as osteocytes. These spaces are called lacunae. Radiating from all directions from the lacunae are small channels known as canaliculi.

These small channels (canaliculi) are filled with extracellular fluid and contain finger-like processes of the osteocytes. The canaliculi connect lacunae with each other and with the central canals. This intricate branching network provides many routes for blood-borne nutrients and oxygen to diffuse through the fluid to the osteocytes and for wastes to diffuse back into the blood. Areas between the Haversian systems (osteons) contain what is known as interstitial lamellae, which also have lacunae and canaliculi. These sections are incomplete remains of older osteons.

Cancellous bones consist of lamellae that are arranged in an irregular lattice of thin columns of bone called trabeculae.

The macroscopic spaces between trabeculae of some bones are filled with red bone marrow which produces blood cells. Within the trabeculae are osteocytes in lacunae and radiating from the lacunae are canaliculi.

Bone formation

Bones form in one of two ways. A small number of bones develop on or within fibrous connective tissue membrane through a process known as intra-membranous ossification. Ossification refers to the process by which bone is formed. Bones which develop in this way include the flat bones of the skull, the mandible and the clavicle. However, most bones of the body develop through a process known as endochondral ossification, where the bones develop within hyaline cartilage (Tortora, 2005).

Bone formation involves the activity of cells known as osteoblasts. These cells are found typically in the medullary canal of long bones and under the periosteum. Cells known as osteoclasts are involved in the removal and breakdown of bone.

The human skeleton consists of 206 bones which are grouped into two divisions – the axial skeleton and the appendicular skeleton.

Axial skeleton

These are bones around the axis of the body, of which there are 80 in total.

The bones of the skull are divided into two groups – the bones of the face (14) and the bones of the cranium (8). A suture is an immovable joint found between the bones of the cranium. There are four prominent cranial sutures, namely the coronal, sagittal, lambdoid and squamous (Tortora and Grabowski, 2004).

The vertebral column (spine) has several functions, including enclosing and protecting the spinal cord, supporting the head, giving attachment for ribs and back muscles, protecting the brain from vertical shock, and the presence of intervertebral discs act as shock absorbers. The vertebral column also allows for some movement of the head and trunk.

 Revision Point

The vertebral column is divided into five regions. Name these regions and state how many bones are found in each.

Intervertebral discs are found between the vertebrae from the second cervical to the sacrum. These discs have an outer ring of fibro-cartilage and a soft and pulpy inner core (Tortora and Grabowski, 2004). Intervertebral discs contribute to the flexibility of the vertebral column and as stated above also act as shock absorbers.

The thoracic cage protects the vital organs found within the thorax (chest), and is made up from the thoracic vertebrae, the ribs and the sternum (breastbone). There are 12 pairs of ribs, and the sternum is divided into 3 parts – the manubrium, the body and the xiphoid process.

Appendicular skeleton

This refers to the appendages and girdles and amounts in total to 126 bones.

The shoulder girdle consists of two bones – the scapula (shoulder blade) and the clavicle (collar bone). The bones of the upper extremities consist of the humerus, the radius and ulna, the carpals and the metacarpals and phalanges.

The pelvic girdle consists of three bones – the ileum, the ischium and the pubis. The bones of the lower extremities consist of the femur, the tibia and fibula, the tarsals and the metatarsals and phalanges.

Joints

A joint or articulation is the point of contact between bones, or between cartilage and bones. They are classified by two methods. One is to classify according to the degree of movement allowed by the joint, where some permit no movement between the articulating bones, some permit slight movement and others permit a great deal of movement. The other way to classify them is dependent upon their structure, that is, whether they have a joint space between the articulating bones and what kind of support tissue binds the bones together (Tortora, 2005). Based on the structure, there are three types of joints in the body – fibrous, cartilaginous and synovial.

A fibrous joint lacks a joint cavity and the bones are united by fibrous connective tissue. Generally, they are immovable joints in the adult, although some allow slight movement. Examples include the sutures between bones of the skull, and the joints between the teeth and upper and lower jaw (maxilla and mandible).

A cartilaginous joint lacks a joint cavity and the bones are unified by a plate of hyaline cartilage. They permit little or no movement. Examples include the symphysis pubis and the joints between the bodies of the vertebral bones.

A synovial joint has a joint cavity present. The bone ends are covered with smooth hyaline cartilage. The joint is lubricated by a thick fluid called synovial fluid and is enclosed by a flexible articular capsule, which may be supported by ligaments. These joints allow a great deal of movement. Examples include the hip, knee, shoulder and elbow.

Skeletal muscle

Skeletal muscle is responsible for movement, maintaining body posture and heat production within the body.

 Revision Point

Name the four major functional characteristics of skeletal muscle that play an important role in the maintenance of homeostasis.

Control of skeletal muscles

Skeletal muscle are under voluntary control. Their fibres normally contract only when sufficient stimulus is applied by a nerve ending. Nerves that innervate skeletal muscle divide into several branches before they terminate. Each branch is then distributed to an individual muscle fibre. In this way, a nerve impulse passing along a neurone will result in the simultaneous contraction of all the muscle fibres which are innervated by that particular nerve cell. A group of muscle fibres that receive their innervation from a single neurone is called a motor unit. An individual muscle may contain hundreds or thousands of individual motor units.

A lever system

Bones work as a system of levers, and muscles provide the power to make them move. A skeletal muscle is attached to one bone at one end of a joint, travels across the joint and is then connected to another bone at the other end of the joint. When the muscle contracts, one bone is pulled towards the other.

Posture

The upright posture is maintained by the simultaneous contraction of appropriate sets of muscles. However, not every muscle is required to continually contract in order to maintain posture. In this way, energy is saved, as we are not using the whole muscle (sets of muscle). Energy expenditure in maintaining posture is reduced by other means too:

- As already stated, we use only a part of each muscle – the postural tension of a muscle is maintained by only a small number of its fibres, and these fibres are constantly changing, resulting in the minimising of fatigue.
- We use ligaments – ligaments either within or outwith a joint help to hold the joint in place and give general support to the joint.
- Balance – when standing in a balanced position, the joints are in their most stable position and minimal muscular energy is required to maintain the posture. Standing off balance puts the body in an unstable position and more muscular energy is required in order to remain upright.

Ageing changes related to mobilising

Bones

The bones, joints and muscles are all affected by changes caused by the ageing process. These changes have a significant effect on the quality of older people's lives as they can have a considerable effect on functional ability and can impact negatively on the level of independence in older people (Roach, 2001).

The relationship between bone formation and bone absorption is dynamic over the lifespan of an individual. Bone formation (osteoblast activity) exceeds the bone absorption (osteoclast activity) rate during the period from birth to adolescence, but then bone formation and absorption equalise during the twenties. However, with advancing age, the rate of bone absorption changes. Around the age of 30, bone absorption starts to surpass bone formation. From this age, there is a steady and progressive decrease in cancellous bone loss beginning in the thirties and continuing into old age (Matteson et al., 1997).

Cancellous bone loss starts before compact bone loss and the ratio of compact bone to cancellous bone increases with age. By the age of 80, men will lose ∼27% of cancellous bone, whereas women will lose ∼43% of cancellous bone by the age of 90. With the onset of the menopause, there is a sharp increase in cancellous bone loss due to the loss of protection from the hormone oestrogen. Compact bone loss occurs from the age of 45 in women and the age of 50 in men. Not only does compact bone loss occur at an earlier age in women, it also occurs at a faster rate than in men (Matteson et al., 1997). A vast amount of cancellous bone is found in the vertebral bodies, wrist and hip. Consequently, older people are at increased risk of sustaining fractures in all of those areas (Roach, 2001).

Other changes related to the bones occur through the ageing process, including a decrease in height with age and a change in posture as an older adult may become more stooped. Height decrease is more commonly found in women than in men although it occurs in both sexes (Matteson et al., 1997). As much as 1–6 inches (2.5–15 cm) can be lost in height. Shortening of the spinal column results in what is commonly called a dowager's hump, that is, kyphosis of the upper thoracic spine. These changes are related to loss of fluid in the fibro-cartilage within the intervertebral discs. As a consequence of this fluid loss, the fibro-cartilage becomes drier, thinner and more delicate. This increases the risk of tearing and contributes to vertebral compression and a decrease in a person's height. As a result of the shortening of the spinal column, a person's arms and legs can appear to be longer, although there is no change in their length. Accompanying the changes in the fibro-cartilage, bony outgrowths called osteophytes develop on the vertebral column. These growths are typical of changes associated with osteoarthritis. Osteophytes can also develop on the articulating surfaces of bones making up joints. Within these joints, smooth, articular cartilage may be replaced by a rougher cartilage. The cartilage can also become thicker with advancing age and lose some of its elasticity (Timiras, 2003).

The lordotic curve which can be found in the lower back flattens, and both flexion and extension of the lower back are decreased (Lueckenotte, 2000). A combination of all of the bone changes, including increased flexion of the hips and knees, decreased lumbar lordosis, increased thoracic kyphosis and rounded shoulders with protracted scapula impact on and lead to the familiar stooped posture. The stooped posture can lead to the head jutting forward and tilting upward to maintain gaze level. The individual's centre of gravity is affected and a slower, shorter, more cautious and wider based gait pattern is developed in old age (MacAnaw, 2001). There are slight differences in the gait changes for men and women. In men, the gait becomes small stepped with a wider based stance. Women become bow legged with a narrower standing base, and walk with a waddling gait (Lueckenotte, 2000).

Activity

Using observation, how many of the above changes can you identify in your clients when they are mobilising.

Increased bone re-absorption has an impact on the amount of calcium in the body. The bone loses calcium and the ability to produce material for the bone matrix is diminished. This results in weakening of the intracellular bone, causing bone to become weaker, thus increasing the risk of fracture for older people (Roach, 2001). The recommended daily intake of calcium for younger adults is between 800 and 1300 mg, and 1200 mg daily for adults over 51 years of age (Maher et al., 2002). Also associated with advancing age is a decreased proficiency in the ability of the body to absorb calcium from the digestive system (Matteson et al., 1997).

In some older women, parathyroid hormone levels increase with ageing, but the contribution of this increase to bone loss may be minimal. The increase in parathyroid levels may represent a compensatory response to reduced intestinal absorption of calcium and subsequent low plasma calcium levels (Timiras, 2003). Vitamin D manufacture in the skin may also be affected if an older person is housebound and unable to venture outside due to reduced mobility, and this will further impact on any dietary deficiencies of calcium.

Activity

Identify foods and fluids which are rich in calcium and vitamin D. How much of each identified food/fluid would an older person have to take in order to achieve their recommended daily amount?

Physical activity increases stress and strain on the skeleton due to muscular contraction and gravity. It improves blood flow to exercising muscles and indirectly increases venous return. Physical activity involving weight loading also stimulates build up of bone minerals. Physical activity includes gentle exercise such as walking and dancing. Engaging in such activities will not only provide a cardiovascular workout for the individual, but also encourage mineralisation of bones as identified earlier. An accumulation of 30 minutes of moderate activity on most days of the week is recommended by the Scottish Government (2006).

Joints

The effects of ageing are most commonly felt in the freely movable synovial joints including the knees, wrists, elbows and hips. The synovial membrane which lines the joint cavity secretes a lubricating fluid called synovial fluid. As ageing progresses, the amount of synovial fluid secreted diminishes. The articular cartilage which lines the joint surfaces reduces friction within the joint and also acts as a shock absorber. With advancing age, the cartilage frays, thins and erodes, so that the bones may come into direct contact with each other (MacAnaw, 2001). The ligaments also lose their elasticity so that they shorten and become less flexible. The resultant changes lead to a reduced range of movement in the affected joints (Roach, 2001).

Muscles

The major function of skeletal muscle is to provide the power to allow bones to move. Muscle strength reaches a peak between the ages of 20 and 30 and starts to decline during middle age. This decline continues at a more or less constant rate as we age, irrespective of the muscle group considered. By the age of 80, ~50% of maximum muscle mass is lost (Roach, 2001). However, the rate of decline among muscle groups is variable. The diaphragm remains active throughout life and undergoes little change with ageing. In contrast, the soleus muscle of the leg shows reduced strength with ageing. However, it is possible to increase skeletal muscle power by physical training, even in old age (McMurdo, 2000). Thus, this ageing change is not only reversible, it is also preventable.

The number of muscle fibres reduces with age, resulting in a loss of lean body mass (Roach, 2001). This loss of body mass is known as sarcopenia and results in muscle weakness (Timiras, 2003). Muscles of the lower extremities seem to atrophy more and lose more strength than upper extremity muscles. This may be due to the upper extremity muscles being used more frequently for day-to-day living (MacAnaw, 2001).

Muscle tissue regenerates more slowly with advancing age and tissue that is atrophied is replaced with fibrous tissue. This effect can be seen quite clearly when looking at the muscles of the hands, as they become thin and bony, with deep inter-osseous spaces.

Changes in both the musculoskeletal and the nervous systems result in slower movement (Matteson et al., 1997). This occurs because the density of blood vessel capillaries per motor unit diminishes with age, whereas oxygen utilisation per motor unit remains steady. Muscle contraction slows as the result of prolonged impulse conduction time along the motor unit in muscle tissue (Matteson et al., 1997). Increased muscle rigidity contributes to limited movement in areas such as the neck, shoulder, hips and knees (Roach, 2001). The degree of muscle rigidity can be assessed by measuring the amount of resistance to passive movement.

A decline in muscle mass may parallel the decline in muscle strength, but it does not affect endurance. Endurance can be maintained in older age because type 1 muscle fibres do not atrophy with age. Type 1 muscle fibres are slower contracting fibres. High speed performance is affected by type 2 muscle fibres, which are the fast contracting fibres. Ageing athletes are therefore better able to compete in endurance events, rather than events where there are bursts of speed required.

There are significant amounts of lipofuscin (age-related waste material) and fat deposited within skeletal muscle tissue. Skeletal muscle loses the usual red brown colour due to the loss of myoglobin pigment and they become yellow due to the increased deposition of lipofuscin pigment and fat cells (Matteson et al., 1997).

In order to remain balanced, older people require posture and moving equipoise. Balance is the ability to stand steadily, posture is the alignment of body segments in proper relation to one another and moving equipoise is the control of equilibrium in movements (Linton and Matteson, 1997). Information about the length, tension and speed of muscle activity is provided by muscle spindle and tendon proprioception. This can be described as muscle joint sense and is monitored within the brain. The brain responds to these stimuli by bringing about actions which help to maintain balance, posture and controlled integration of movements. In this way, the body responds appropriately to stimuli in order to maintain correct balance and position.

Control of posture diminishes with age, as a result of a decrease in sensory cues from proprioceptors, declining function of stretch reflexes that initiate from muscle spindles and slower processing of information in the brain. Older people come to depend on visual control to maintain postural stability and visual acuity decreases with advancing age.

Postural sway also increases with age. This change affects women more noticeably than men (Matteson et al., 1997).

Age-related health problems

Osteoporosis

Osteoporosis is a metabolic bone disorder where the balance between bone breakdown and bone build up is lost; that is more bone is broken down (re-absorbed) than is built up. This leads to a reduction in bone mass which typically affects the trabeculae without there being a deficit in bone mineralisation. This contributes to the fragility of bones. The bones become lighter and weaker with thinner cortical bone, less trabeculae and widening of the medullary canal. These weaker, brittle bones are therefore susceptible to fracture.

Oestrogen and testosterone encourage osteoblast activity and synthesis of bone matrix (Tortora, 2005). Oestrogen levels decrease significantly in women at menopause which accelerates the rate of bone loss, whereas levels of testosterone in men only decrease slightly with age. In females, the level of cytokines rises as the levels of oestrogen falls, resulting in increased activity of osteoclasts which break down bone tissue.

Risk factors for the development of osteoporosis include genetic factors, decreasing oestrogen hormone levels at and post menopause, age as bone mineral density decreases with advancing age, gender with women more likely to develop osteoporosis as they have less bone mass compared to men and their bones are smaller than men's bones (SIGN 71, 2003). Smoking, low BMI, poor intake of calcium and vitamin D and low levels of weight-bearing exercise, all contribute to the development of osteoporosis. Dietary calcium and vitamin D intake must be adequate to maintain bone remodelling and body functions. Vitamin D is necessary for the absorption of calcium and for normal bone mineralisation. Inadequate intake of calcium or vitamin D over a period of years results in decreased bone mass. Weight-bearing exercise slows the rate at which bone mineral density is reduced.

Normal bone remodelling in the adult results in increased bone mass until about the age of 30 (Huether and McCance, 2004). Genetic factors, nutrition, lifestyle choices and physical activity all influence the timing of peak bone mass. Age-related loss begins soon after peak bone mass is achieved.

With osteoporosis, there can be a gradual collapse of spinal vertebrae over a period of time, which may be asymptomatic. This can be observed as progressive kyphosis (increased curvature of the thoracic vertebrae). With the development of kyphosis, there is an associated loss of height.

Assessment and diagnosis

Bone mineral density is the principal measure for the diagnosis and ongoing monitoring of osteoporosis (SIGN 71, 2003). Dual-energy X-ray absorptiometry (DEXA) scans are considered the gold standard for diagnosis of osteoporosis and are used to measure bone mineral density. Sites used to measure bone mineral density include the lumbar spine, the hip and the wrist. SIGN 71 (2003) advise using two separate sites and indicate their preference as the spine and the hip.

Management

Management goals are to prevent osteoporosis, arrest or slow the process down and relieve existing symptoms. Prevention begins early with the identification and education of people at risk. Adequate dietary and/or supplemental calcium, regular weight-bearing exercise and modification of lifestyle all help to maintain bone mass. Weight-bearing exercise should target the spine and hip as these are the two sites commonly affected by osteoporosis (Walker, 2008). Simply going for regular walks can reduce the risk of hip fractures in post-menopausal women (Feskanich et al., 2002).

Calcium and vitamin D intake should be monitored and supplements used where appropriate. Outdoor activities with exposure to sunlight can help as vitamin D is produced by skin in response to exposure to ultraviolet radiation from natural sunlight.

A number of drugs are available that influence bone mineral density, including bisphosphonates, calcitonin, strontium ranelate, teriparatide and raloxifene. All these drugs help to reduce the risk of fracture in post-menopausal women (Walker, 2008).

Falls in older people

Falls are not an inevitable consequence of ageing; however, the physical and psychological effects of falls can be wide ranging and potentially serious, if not fatal. Thirty per cent of adults over 65 who live in the community and 50% of those over 80 will fall over a 12-month period, while 60% of those who fall once, fall again within the same year (Oliver, 2007). Oliver goes on to state after falling many older adults find it difficult to rise from the ground, resulting in a lengthy period of immobility which can lead to hypothermia, dehydration and pressure area damage.

Older people are also much more likely to die after a fall than younger people because of the risk of fractures and head injuries. Over 90% of fractures results from falls. Approximately 25% of falls, where there is direct impact on the trochanteric area of the hip, result in a fracture. In the hospital setting, ~10% of patients who have fallen will die before discharge (Tideiksaar, 1998). According to Holmes (2006), an older person in the United Kingdom dies every 5 hours as a result of a fall at home. The psychological fear of falling can also have a detrimental effect on an older person's daily activities (Bazian, 2005) and their overall quality of life. A fall can lead to loss of confidence and increasing anxiety for both the older person who falls and their carer (Oliver, 2007).

A fall can be defined as 'an unexpected, involuntary loss of balance by which a person comes to rest at a lower or ground level' (Commodore, 1995). Falls are under-reported as people are ashamed of falling or they are unwilling to admit that they have fallen. They may also think that falling is a consequence of growing older. The term fall is now viewed as a contentious word, as it is perceived to be associated with people who are old, frail and dependant (DH, 2001). Falls in older people should be taken seriously as they may indicate underlying health or social problems.

Causes

The causes of falls are many and varied and have traditionally been divided into intrinsic and extrinsic factors. However, this distinction may not always be useful as falls tend to be multifactorial. In other words, there is normally more than one reason for a fall. Falls are often related to the multifactorial relationship between several risk factors, the external environment and the older person's own activities and awareness or attitudes to risk. A trip or a fall may be a combination of both intrinsic and extrinsic factors, for example, someone trips over their rug but this may not have happened if their eyesight had been better or they were not hurrying (Oliver, 2007). The descriptions older people use to describe an event is important as they may not have used the word fall but use other descriptions including a slip, trip or an accident (Kelly and Dowling, 2004). The meaning that an older person ascribes to a fall will influence whether they report the fall. Table 9.1 lists the most common factors that are implicated in falls.

However, some of the factors require further explanation. Older people are rarely asked about their alcohol intake and they may have a higher weekly intake than is recommended for a number of reasons, including loneliness or bereavement. There is a range of medications that commonly increase the incidence of falls and they include centrally sedating agents such as sedatives, hypnotics, opiates and anticonvulsants. Drugs that can precipitate postural hypotension such as anti-hypertensives, anti-arrhythmics and diuretics may also increase the incidence of falls (Oliver, 2007). In hospital, the use of bed rails increase the risk of falls as patients may try to 'escape' the confines of their bed by climbing over, under or through the bed rails.

The ageing changes related to falls not only involve musculoskeletal changes, but also changes in vision and hearing (see Chapter 4). The ability to maintain balance requires the constant interaction of three fundamental processes: (i) recognition via sensory nerves, for example, eyesight, touch and proprioception (a sense of where the body is in space and where the various parts of the body are located in relation to each other), (ii) interpretation of theses impulses in the CNS and (iii) adjustment via motor nerves such as reflexes, conscious movement and muscular contraction. If one or more of these processes are impaired, then the risk of fall increases (Oliver, 2007).

Table 9.1 Common factors implicated in falls. (Reproduced from Oliver (2007). With permission.)

Intrinsic factors	Extrinsic factors
Acute illness	Physical environment
Changes in vision	Inadequate footwear
Changes in balance	Unsuitable walking aids
Cardiovascular changes	Poor ambient lighting
Neurological disease	Visual contrasts between surfaces
Medications	Dirty or ineffective spectacles and loose mats
Alcohol intake (Kelly and Dowling, 2004)	Slippery surfaces
	Trailing cables
	Pets
	Difficult stairs or access; inappropriate bed, chair or toilet seat height for safe transfer

Where vision is concerned, the lens becomes less flexible as we grow older so that the eye does not accommodate so readily. This is described as presbyopia. Presbyopia can affect depth perception so that when a person is going up or down stairs, it may be difficult for them to judge accurately the depth of steps, which can increase their likelihood of stumbling and falling. Advice here is to use a banister (hand rail) and not to rush. Vision can also be affected by eye glare if a cataract is forming/has formed. Being outside on sunny days or indoors when bright lights shine on polished floor surfaces can also increase the risk of falls due to glare (Kelly and Dowling, 2004).

Changes in the ear include atrophy of the ossicles (malleus, incus and stapes) in the middle ear which causes changes in sound conduction resulting in the potential loss of high tone frequencies. This is called presbycusis. Background noise is amplified and there is a decrease in directional hearing. This decrease in directional hearing increases the risk of falls as it can be disorientating to the person, who can be startled by sudden and unexpected noises.

In the cardiovascular system, the loss of tissue elasticity in arteries leads to a decrease in tissue recoil, resulting in changes in blood pressure with alterations in body position. As a result, older adults who lie flat and rise up suddenly are more likely to experience a drop in blood pressure and a feeling of light-headedness due to this loss of tissue elasticity and recoil. There is also an overall reduction in reaction time which makes it more difficult for older people to correct themselves before they fall (Kelly and Dowling, 2004).

 Point for Practice

Review your own area of clinical practice and identify potential hazards which may contribute to increasing the risk of falls in your client group.

Falls risk assessment

The NICE (2004) guidelines identify the main areas of assessment that require consideration when assessing older adults for their risk in relation to falling. They identify that multifactorial assessment should include the following areas:

- Identification of falls history.
- Assessment of gait, balance and mobility, and muscle weakness.
- Assessment of osteoporosis risk.
- Assessment of the older persons' perceived functional ability and fear of falling.
- Assessment of visual impairment.
- Assessment of cognitive impairment and neurological examination.
- Assessment of urinary incontinence.
- Cardiovascular examination and medication review.

Kelly and Dowling (2004) suggest that the identification of a falls history should also include a description of symptoms before the fall, including feelings of dizziness and palpitations and whether the legs gave way from under them. Blood pressure and pulse should be monitored and ECG may be taken if the fall is unexplained.

Older people who are unsteady when they stand up from a chair without the use of their arms require further assessment and high-risk groups require a comprehensive detailed assessment (AGS et al., 2001).

The hospital setting should also be considered when assessing a person for the risk of falls. These should include how long the patient has been in hospital, time of day when a fall occurred and number of nursing staff on duty at that time (Kelly and Dowling, 2004).

There are a number of available risk assessment tools but they will normally incorporate most, if not all, of the suggestions put forward by NICE (2004). The Cannard risk assessment tool is an example of one such tool (Figure 9.1).

Circle all options which apply to the person. Put the score for each topic in the right-hand box. Add all the scores in the right-hand boxes and put the total in the grand total box. The maximum possible score is 32. Some topics have more than one scorable option – score all that apply. The final score is necessary to know how to proceed when following the Falls Guidelines.

Scores: 3–8 = low risk   9–12 = medium risk   13+ = high risk.

Interventions

Multifactorial interventions including strength and balance training have been shown to decrease the risk of falls in older adults. Those most likely to benefit from these interventions are older people living at home with a history of recurrent falls and/or balance and gait deficit (NICE, 2004). An individualised programme should be initiated and closely followed and monitored by an appropriately trained professional. An exercise programme is also recommended for older people in long-term care settings who are at risk of falling.

Home hazard assessment/intervention also reduces the risk of falls. Older people who have received treatment in hospital after a fall should be offered a home hazard assessment and safety interventions/modifications by a suitably trained health professional, for example an occupational therapist. These visits will highlight possible risks at home and interventions targeted to overcome these risks should be implemented.

Activity
Given the opportunity, you should try to accompany an occupational therapist when on a home visit with a client.

Older people identified at risk from falls should also have a thorough vision assessment and be referred to an optician/ophthalmologist for corrective treatment. Review of current medications should be a priority for older adults at risk from falling. Pharmacist inclusion is of paramount importance, where a thorough review and modification/removal of medications, including over-the-counter drugs, is undertaken.

Cannard Risk	No.	1	2	3	4	5	6	7	8	9	10
	Initials										
Assessment	Date										
SEX											
Male	1										
Female	2										
AGE											
60–70	1										
71–80	2										
81+	1										
SENSORY DEFICIT											
None	0										
Hearing Deficit	1										
Sight Deficit	2										
Balance Deficits	2										
FALLS HISTORY											
None	0										
In Ward	1										
At Home	2										
Both	3										
MEDICATION TYPE											
None	0										
Sleeping Tablets	1										
Hypotensives	1										
Tranquilisers	1										
MEDICAL HISTORY											
None	0										
Diabetes	1										
Fits	1										
Confusion	1										
MOBILITY											
Bed Bound	1										
Fully Mobile	1										
Uses Aid	2										
Restricted	3										
GAIT											
Steady	0										
Hesitant In Initiating Movement	1										
Poor Transfer	3										
Unsteady	3										
TOTAL SCORE											

Figure 9.1   Cannard risk assessment tool. (Reproduced from Cannard (1996). With permission.)

The use of walking aids should be included as an intervention in relation to reducing risk of falls. Proper training in their use can help maintain confidence when mobilising and assist with maintenance of independence.

Education

The frequency of falls can be decreased and may be prevented by implementing a number of simple measures identified by NICE (2004) which are outlined below:

- Following a home hazard assessment/intervention visit, implement specific measures to reduce risk and prevent falls.
- Give information and support regarding motivation with continuation of prevention strategies to reduce risk of falling. This will include exercise and balancing training.
- Discuss the preventable nature of some falls with your client.
- Offer discussion about the physical and psychological benefits of modifying falls risk for example reduced anxiety and increased confidence when mobilising. Improved muscle tone which adds to confidence and ability when mobilising.
- Offer advice in relation to where further information may be sought for example age concern or help the aged.
- Identify coping strategies if a fall occurs, including getting back up after a fall and how to summon help if unable to rise.
- Consider the use of hip protectors where appropriate. However, there is little evidence that they are useful in preventing fractures after a fall. They may, however, improve confidence when mobilising.

(Adapted from NICE, 2004)

The use of hip protectors may be useful in allowing older people to feel safer when mobilising and reduce the fear of falling (Hill and Schwartz, 2004). However, for maximum protection, they should be worn 24 hours per day. The need to wear these protectors for 24 hours a day reduces patient concordance.

Preventative measures

For people who have been identified as at risk from falls, pads containing alarms are available which detect movement from a lying position to a more upright position. This informs others of a person's movements and therefore alerts carers to the possibility of a fall. Preventative measures can then be implemented to reduce this risk.

A person's physical environment can be modified to reduce the risk of falls. Simple measures such as application of anti-skid wax on floors, use of non-skid rugs and the wearing of low-heeled shoes with good traction can all reduce the risk of falls.

Remember that restraints such as bed rails can do more harm than good as people may fall from a greater height as they attempt to climb over the bed rail. Pillows under mattresses may be used to prevent people from rolling out of bed. If a person is deemed to be at considerable risk from falling from their bed, they can be managed on a mattress on the floor. This is a safe and accepted practice to engage in (Tideiksaar, 1998).

Key points from NICE (2004) guidelines on falls prevention in older people:

- Health-care professionals should regularly ask their clients if they have fallen.
- Older people who have fallen, had recurrent falls or are at risk of falling should receive: multifactorial risk assessment, individualised multifactorial interventions and strength and balance training.
- Home hazard assessment with safety modifications should be given after hospital discharge following a fall.
- Participation in falls prevention programme should be encouraged.
- Psychotropic medications should be reviewed and stopped if possible.
- Cardiac pacing should be considered for people with heart problems and unexplained falls.

Where falls cannot be completely prevented, it is often possible to minimise the consequences, using measure such as environmental modifications as discussed previously, bone strengthening drugs such as bisphosphonates if at risk from osteoporosis or diagnosed with osteoporosis and the use of community alarms to alert others of a fall whilst at home.

There is an expectation that there will be falls amongst older adults in a clinical area. Zero falls may indicate that older people are over protected and cocooned by carers to the point where their quality of life can be diminished. Despite having preventative measures in place to reduce the risk of falls, older people are entitled to take risks associated with mobilising.

Exercise

As with younger individuals, engagement in a regular exercise programme has many benefits for older people and is associated with longevity and enhanced well-being (Aranceta et al., 2001). Older adults can be advised to participate in such programmes which should be devised to encourage active participation and maximise enjoyment. If people enjoy participation in exercise, it is likely that they will remain involved and not opt out from these activities. Physical inactivity has been linked with muscle atrophy, decreased endurance, a reduction in muscle strength and an increased likelihood of falls (Thomson, 2002). Physical activity enhances muscle strength and joint flexibility, both of which help preserve mobility. Exercise also reduces the risk of falls by enhancing agility (Meiner and Lueckenotte, 2006). Given the outcomes of physical inactivity, any movement is of benefit and all older adults should be encouraged to engage in exercise, no matter how little or infrequent.

According to Mauk (2006), direct benefits of exercise include a reduction in resting blood pressure, an improvement in cholesterol levels, better control of diabetes mellitus and enhanced cognitive functioning. Indirectly, exercise also enhances sleep, mood and general well-being. Jones and Jones (1997) also suggest that exercise reduces the risk of heart disease and osteoporosis. Blood pressure can also be reduced, weight controlled and sleep enhanced. Aerobic exercise such as brisk walking reduces low-density lipoprotein (LDL) levels and raises high-density lipoprotein (HDL) levels (Halm and Penque, 1999). Remember that LDLs are referred to as 'bad' cholesterol and can slowly build up in the inner walls of arteries, contributing to the development of atherosclerosis and increasing the risk of cardiovascular disease. HDLs or 'good' cholesterol reduces the risk of cardio-vascular disease.

Prior to embarking upon an exercise programme, it is advisable for the older adult to discuss this with their GP. A routine physical examination may also be in order.

Mazzeo and Tanaka (2001) suggest that an exercise programme for older adults should include the following:

- A period of warm-up activities including gentle stretching of muscles.
- Exercise should be of low to moderate intensity rather than vigorous and intense.
- A minimum of 30 minutes low intensity exercise should be performed, preferably on a daily basis. If an individual cannot participate in exercise for 30 minutes duration, three intervals of 10 minutes low intensity exercise is also beneficial. If more exercise is desired, the individual is encouraged to increase the duration rather than the intensity of exercise.
- The type of exercise engaged in should be determined by interest, availability and fitness levels. Cycling, walking and swimming are all beneficial.

Older adults should be reminded to maintain levels of hydration before, during and after exercise. Fluids should be taken regularly as body fluids will be lost during exercise (Meiner and Lueckenotte, 2006). It might be appropriate to exercise with a partner. This can help with motivation to exercise and can add to the overall enjoyment and safety during exercise. If chest pain or tightness, shortness of breath, dizziness or palpitations are experienced during exercise, the person should be advised to stop and seek help immediately (Meiner and Lueckenotte, 2006).

Exercises in water (aquatic therapy) are particularly effective in improving balance and increasing the strength and range of motion. Movement within the water is enhanced, flexibility is increased and pain experienced during exercise is reduced. Aquatic therapy may enhance balance and stability which inturn may reduce the risk of falls.

Structured physical therapy benefits older frail persons living in care settings. Exercising in this formal manner helps older adults with their physical impairments and enhances musculoskeletal function (Mauk, 2006). Yoga can also improve movement in the older adult. The risk of falls may be reduced by enhancing an older person's muscular strength, balance and stamina.

In order to increase the levels of exercise engaged upon, it may take nothing more than advising older adults to leave their car a little further away from where they are going than normal or to walk up stairs rather than take the elevator or escalator, especially if only going up one or two flights of stairs. As stated previously, a little exercise is better than none and it all adds up in the end.

Summary

It is important that as we age we stay physically active. Movement and activity help to ensure the health of most, if not all, body systems. Inactivity carries life-limiting and life-threatening risks. Whilst a certain amount of wear and tear is a normal consequence of ageing, this should not necessarily limit an older person's mobility.

Ageing carries two risks in particular that are explored within this chapter, namely osteoporosis and the risk of falling. Once again, we see the importance of the health-care professional in relation to adequate assessment and prevention of these risks.

References and further reading

American Geriatrics Society, British Geriatrics Society and American Academy of Orthopaedic Surgeons Panel on Falls Prevention. 2001. Guideline for the prevention of falls in older persons. Journal of the American Geriatrics Society 49(5), 664–672.

Aranceta, J., Perez-Rodrigo, C., Gondra, J. and Orduna, J. 2001. Community-based programme to promote physical activity among elderly people: the GeroBilbo study. The Journal of Nutrition, Health and Aging 5, 238–242.

Bazian Ltd. 2005. Fall prevention programmes in older people. Evidence-Based Healthcare and Public Health 9, 343–348.

Cannard, G. 1996. Falling trend. Nursing Times 92(2), 36–37.

Commodore, D. 1995. Falls in the elderly population: a look at the incidence, risks, healthcare costs, and preventative strategies. Rehabilitation Nursing 20(2), 84–89.

Department of Health. 2001. The National Service Framework for Older People. The Stationary Office, London.

Feskanich, D., Willett, W. and Colditz, G. 2002. Walking and leisure-time activity and risk of hip fracture in post-menopausal women. Journal of the American Medical Association 288(18), 2300–2306.

Halm, M. and Penque, S. 1999. Heart disease in women. American Journal of Nursing 99(4), 26.

Hill, K. and Schwartz, J. 2004. Assessment and management of falls in older people. International Medicine Journal 34, 557–564.

Holmes, P. 2006. Supporting older people: promoting falls prevention. British Journal of Community Nursing 11(6), 247–248, 250.

Huether, S.E. and McCance, K.L. 2004. Understanding Pathophysiology. 3rd ed. Mosby, St. Louis, MO.

Jones, J. and Jones, K.D. 1997. Promoting physical activity in the senior years. Journal of Gerontological Nursing 23(7), 40.

Kelly, A. and Dowling, M. 2004. Reducing the likelihood of falls in older people. Nursing Standard 18(49), 33–40.

Lueckenotte, A.G. 2000. Gerontologic Nursing. 2nd ed. Mosby, St. Louis, MO.

Linton, A. and Matteson, M. 1997. Age related changes in the neurological system. In Matteson, M., McConnell, E. and Linton, A. (Eds). Gerontological Nursing. Concepts and Practice. 2nd ed. WB Saunders Company, Philadelphia, PA.

MacAnaw, M. 2001. Normal changes with aging. In Maas, M., Buckwalter, K., Hardy, M., Tripp-Reimer, T., Titler, M. and Specht, J.P. (Eds). Nursing Care of Older Adults: Diagnoses, Outcomes and Interventions. Mosby, St. Louis, MO.

Maher, A.B., Salmond, S.W. and Pellino, T.A. 2002. Orthopaedic Nursing. 3rd ed. WB Saunders, Philadelphia, PA.

Matteson, M., McConnell, E. and Linton, A. 1997. Gerontological Nursing: Concepts and Practice. 2nd ed. WB Saunders, Philadelphia, PA.

Mauk, K.L. 2006. Gerontological Nursing: Competencies for Care. Jones and Bartlett Publishers, Sudbury, MA.

Mazzeo, R.S. and Tanaka, H. 2001. Exercise prescription for the elderly: current recommendations. Sports Medicine 31(11), 809–819.

McMurdo, M.E.T. 2000. A healthy old age: realistic or futile goal? British Medical Journal 321(7269), 1149–1151.

Meiner, S.E. and Lueckenotte, A.G. 2006. Gerontologic Nursing. 3rd ed. Mosby Elsevier, St. Louis, MO.

NICE. 2004. Clinical Practice Guideline for the Assessment and Prevention of Falls in Older People. CG21. National Institute for Clinical Excellence, London.

Oliver, D. 2007. Older people who fall: why they matter and what you can do. British Journal of Community Nursing 12(11), 500–507.

Roach, S. 2001. Introductory Gerontological Nursing. Lippincott, Philadelphia, PA.

SIGN. 2003. Management of Osteoporosis. A National Clinical Guideline. 71. Scottish Intercollegiate Guidelines Network, Edinburgh.

Thomson, L.V. 2002. Skeletal muscle adaptations with age, inactivity, and therapeutic physical activity. Journal of Orthopaedic and Sports Physical Therapy 32(2), 44–57.

Tideiksaar, R. 1998. Falls in Older Persons: Prevention and Management. 2nd ed. Health Professions Press, Baltimore, MD.

Timiras, P. 2003. The skeleton, joints and skeletal and cardiac muscles. In Timiras, P. (Ed). Physiological Basis of Aging and Geriatrics. 3rd ed. CRC Press, Boca Raton, FL.

Tortora, G. 2005. Principles of Human Anatomy. 10th ed. Wiley, Hoboken, NJ.

Tortora, G.J. and Grabowski, S.R. 2004. Introduction to the Human Body: Essentials of Anatomy and Physiology. 6th ed. John Wiley & Sons, New Jersey.

Walker, J. 2008. Osteoporosis: pathogenesis, diagnosis and management. Nursing Standard 22(17), 48–56.

Useful websites

Sport, Exercise and Physical Activity: Public Participation, Barriers and Attitudes. www.scotland. gov.uk/Publications/2006/09/29134901/1 – 14 November 2006.

Chapter 10

Expressing Sexuality

Aims

After reading this chapter you will be able to discuss with clients/patients matters related to their sexuality.

Learning Outcomes

After completion of this chapter you will be able to:

- Describe the normal anatomy and functioning of the male and female reproductive tracts
- Conduct a comprehensive patient assessment of the above systems using appropriate tools
- Detail the changes in the above systems that are associated with ageing
- Discuss the presentation and management of some common health problems related to the above systems that occur in older adults.

Introduction

Reflection Point

Consider an older couple known to you. In what ways do they live their 'sexual' selves, that is, express their sexuality?

This chapter will start with an overview of the normal anatomy and physiology of the male and female reproductive systems. We shall then go on to describe the ageing changes throughout both male and female reproductive systems and discuss their effects on the

---

The Physiological Effects of Ageing: Implications for Nursing Practice, First Edition
© Alistair Farley, Ella McLafferty and Charles Hendry
Published 2011 by Blackwell Publishing Ltd

older person's ability to maintain their sexual health. Sexual health assessment tools will be described and analysed in relation to their use with older people before we go on to examine the effects of ageing on the male and female reproductive systems.

Common problems associated with sexual health and older people will be identified, for example this will include problems associated with sexual function, including impotence. We shall discuss the support relating to sexual health that older patients require both in the community and in hospital settings. We shall conclude the chapter by examining the nursing interventions that are required for older adults to attain and maintain adequate sexual health.

Male reproductive system

Normal structure and function

It should be remembered that part of the male reproductive system also forms part of the urinary system. The male reproductive system consists of:

- Reproductive glands: testes (2).
- Ducts for conveying sperm cells: epididymis, vas deferens, ejaculatory duct.
- Associated glands: seminal vesicles, prostate gland, bulbo-urethral glands.
- External genitals: penis.

Testes

The testes (testis – singular) are contained within the scrotum, a pouch of skin and muscle which lies in front of the thighs and behind the penis. Synthesis of sperm requires a temperature cooler than body temperature so the scrotum holds the testes outside the body. Involuntary muscles in the scrotal walls will contract to bring the testes nearer the body if conditions are too cold.

Epididymis

The seminiferous tubules pass to the top of the testes where they unite to form the efferent duct which becomes a single tube called the epididymis. This structure lies coiled and folded down over the back of each testis.

Vas deferens

The epididymis straightens out to form a muscular tube called the vas deferens. The vas is contained within the spermatic cord which also contains the blood vessels, lymph vessels and nerves which supply the testes.

The spermatic cord leaves the scrotum and passes into the abdominal cavity through the inguinal canal. In the abdominal cavity, the vas passes over the ureter and behind the bladder. Here the vas joins the duct from the seminal vesicle to form the ejaculatory duct.

The ejaculatory ducts pass through the prostate gland to enter the urethra.

Prostate gland

This gland surrounds the urethra as it exits the bladder. It is about the size of a golf ball and consists of a fibrous outer capsule surrounding muscular and glandular tissue. Around 45 years of age, the prostate gland typically begins to enlarge (Tortora and Derrickson, 2009). This gland secretes a thin milky fluid that comprises 30% of the volume of semen (Waugh and Grant, 2006). Prostatic fluid provides a supportive and nutritious medium for the transport of sperm. The alkaline nature of prostatic fluid helps to counter the acidic environment of the vagina.

Accessory glands

Other accessory glands associated with the male reproductive system include the seminal vesicles and the bulbo-urethral glands. Seminal vesicles produce semen, a fluid that transports and nourishes sperm after ejaculation (Waugh and Grant, 2006). Similarly, the secretions of the bulbo-urethral glands are alkaline in nature and help to neutralise the acidic environment within the urethra and vagina. They also secrete mucus that helps to lubricate the end of the penis and the lining of the urethra, thus protecting sperm during ejaculation (Tortora and Derrickson, 2009).

Penis

The urethra in the penis forms a common pathway for both urine and semen. The penis consists of three columns of erectile tissue and involuntary muscle well supplied with blood vessels. The columns at the sides of the penis are the corpora cavernosa and the smaller column behind is the corpus spongiosum which contains the urethra. At the end of the penis, the corpus spongiosum extends around the penis to form a bulbous portion called the glans penis. The skin around the glans lies in a loose fold called the foreskin (prepuce). In some men, the foreskin is surgically removed (often in infancy) for religious or health reasons (circumcision).

General function

- The production of spermatozoa (sperm) for fertilisation of the ova.
- Delivery of spermatozoa into the female reproductive system.

Like the female reproductive system, the male reproductive system is regulated by hormones. Male hormones, however, are not secreted in a cyclical fashion. The anterior pituitary gland secretes luteinising hormone (LH) (also called interstitial cell stimulating hormone in males) and follicle stimulating hormone (FSH) in males as well as females.

Interstitial cell stimulating hormone – this hormone causes Leydig cells (interstitial cells) in the testes to secrete testosterone. This hormone is responsible for the development and maintenance of male secondary sexual characteristics. Testosterone also helps in the maturation of seminiferous tubules and regulates the production of sperm (Tortora and Derrickson, 2009; Waugh and Grant, 2006). The secretion of testosterone usually begins to decrease at around the age of 50 (Waugh and Grant, 2006).

Follicle stimulating hormone – this hormone stimulates the production of sperm in the testes.

Unlike in females these hormones are not released in a cyclical fashion, and therefore sperm are produced continuously throughout male adulthood. The production of these hormones is regulated by a negative feedback mechanism.

The production of spermatozoa (**spermatogenesis**) takes place within the seminiferous tubules of the testes, under the influence of these hormones. Primordial germ cells will mature into a primary spermatocyte containing 46 chromosomes. The primary spermatocyte undergoes meiosis (reduction division) to form two secondary spermatocytes, each containing 23 chromosomes. Further division by mitosis produces spermatozoa. Although females produce only one mature ovum per cycle, males produce spermatozoa constantly.

Mature sperm are stored in the epididymis and vas deferens until ejaculation when peristalsis of the sperm ducts carries them out through the urethra in seminal fluid. The total volume of semen in a normal ejaculation is ~2–5 ml, containing about 100 million sperm per ml (Seeley et al., 2005).

Sexual arousal and ejaculation

Male sexual activity occurs in a number of stages. These are:

- Arousal.
- Erection.
- Emission.
- Ejaculation.

Sexual arousal in males is initiated in response to a number of stimuli. Stimuli can be visual, tactile, auditory and olfactory or imagined (Tortora and Derrickson, 2009). These stimuli trigger a response in the hypothalamus. This results in activation of the parasympathetic nervous system. Parasympathetic impulses from the sacral section of the spinal cord initiate and maintain an erection. These impulses cause dilation of arteries supplying the penis. As the penis begins to engorge, the penile veins are compressed, thus obstructing the outflow of blood from the penis. The resulting rise in pressure leads to a rigid, erect penis capable of penetrating the vagina.

With further stimulation, sympathetic nervous activity causes spermatozoa to be propelled from the vas deferens into the prostatic urethra. Furthermore, fluid from the seminal vesicles, bulbo-urethral (Cowper's) gland and prostate is added to form semen. Peristaltic action propels the semen into the penile urethra leading to emission, the discharge of a small volume of semen prior to ejaculation.

Further sympathetic stimulation leads to the contraction of smooth muscle in the urethral wall and of skeletal muscles surrounding the base of the penis (Seeley et al., 2005). Rhythmic contractions force the semen out of the urethra, that is, ejaculation. Just prior to ejaculation, the internal sphincter at the base of the urinary bladder closes preventing semen from entering the bladder. As a result, micturition cannot take place at the same time as ejaculation (Tortora and Derrickson, 2009).

During the sexual act a number of other physiological changes occur, notably an increase in heart rate and blood pressure, increase in respiratory rate and dilation of skin vessels.

Female reproductive system

The female reproductive system consists of a number of internal and external structures, namely:

- Reproductive glands: ovaries (2).
- Uterine or fallopian tubes to carry the ova from the ovaries to the uterus.
- Uterus to contain the developing foetus.
- Vagina through which the male sperm enters the female reproductive tract and the mature foetus is expelled.
- External genitalia.
- Breasts.

Ovaries

The ovaries lie in a shallow depression on the lateral walls of the pelvis (Waugh and Grant, 2006). Each ovary is attached to the uterus by the ovarian ligament and a portion of the broad ligament of the uterus. The ovaries consist of an outer cortex which contains cavities or follicles, each of which contains an immature egg cell or oocyte. These potential egg cells are already present at birth. After puberty, each month one oocyte develops into an ovum and is released from the ovary. This happens under the influence of hormones from the anterior pituitary gland. These hormones, LH and FSH, are released in a cyclical pattern resulting in the menstrual cycle.

The menstrual cycle

Gonadotrophin-releasing hormone (GnRH), secreted by the hypothalamus, regulates the ovarian and uterine cycles. Over a period of 28 days, the cyclical pattern of hormone release brings about a series of changes in the ovaries and uterus called the ovarian or menstrual cycle. FSH stimulates maturation of an ovarian follicle. As it matures, the follicle begins to secrete the hormone oestrogen which further aids the maturation process. LH triggers ovulation, that is, the release of the ovum contained within the follicle. The remaining follicle now forms the corpus luteum. This body begins to secrete progesterone. Progesterone helps to prepare the uterine lining in anticipation of receiving a fertilised ovum for implantation. If fertilisation does not occur, the corpus luteum further degenerates resulting in a fall in hormone levels. Under the influence of falling hormone levels, the uterine lining dies back and sloughs off to be excreted through the vagina resulting in a woman's period, usually lasting 4–5 days. This is the beginning of the next menstrual cycle. The action of oestrogen and progesterone in females is shown in Table 10.1.

Meiosis

Just before ovulation, a primary oocyte (containing 46 chromosomes) undergoes division by meiosis to form two secondary oocytes, each containing 23 chromosomes. Only one of these secondary oocytes will go on to further division by mitosis, resulting in a single mature ovum.

Table 10.1   Action of oestrogen and progesterone.

Oestrogen	Progesterone
Promote development and maintenance of female reproductive structures; secondary sexual characteristics and breasts	Together with oestrogen prepares endometrium for implantation of fertilised ovum
Increase protein metabolism	Prepares breasts for milk secretion
Lower blood cholesterol	High levels inhibit GnRH and LH secretion
Moderate levels inhibit release of GnRH and secretion of LH and FSH	

After the age of 40, menstrual cycles become less regular and eventually cease altogether. This is called the menopause. The low number of follicles which remain in the ovaries are less sensitive to stimulation by LH and FSH, fewer ova are released and levels of oestrogen and progesterone diminish. The menopause is usually complete by the age of 55 (Waugh and Grant, 2006). Once the menopause is complete, a woman is no longer able to conceive naturally.

The fallopian tubes

The ovaries lie at the mouth of the fallopian tubes. These tubes extend laterally from the upper part of the uterus towards the ovaries. The free ends of the tubes are dilated, with finger-like projections called fimbriae. The walls of the tubes contain smooth muscle which is capable of peristalsis, and are lined with ciliated epithelium.

Following ovulation, the released ovum passes into the fimbriae of the fallopian tube and is moved along the tube by peristalsis and the wafting action of the cilia. Fertilisation of the ovum may take place in the fallopian tube if sperm is present.

The uterus

The uterus is a pear-shaped, hollow, muscular organ which lies in the pelvic cavity behind the bladder and in front of the rectum. The upper part of the uterus is the fundus that lies above the openings of the fallopian tubes. The main section of the uterus is known as the body, and the lower part of the uterus is the cervix which extends into the upper part of the vagina.

The uterus is supported in position by ligaments and the pelvic floor muscles. Additionally, support is provided inferiorly by the skeletal muscles of the pelvic floor (Seeley et al., 2005). In some women, the pelvic floor muscles become lax and the uterus slips down into the vagina. This condition is called a uterine prolapse.

The vagina

The vagina is a fibro-muscular tube which connects the internal and external genitalia. The anterior and posterior walls of the vagina lie together in the relaxed state, but the smooth muscle and elastic fibres in the walls allow the vagina to stretch during sexual intercourse and childbirth. The chemical environment in the vagina is acidic due to the presence of lactic acid produced by a bacterium *Lactobacillus acidophilus*. The acidic environment helps to protect the reproductive system from infection. Reduction in the number of these bacilli (such as during treatment with antibiotics) can result in candidiasis infection of the vagina. Although the vaginal walls do not contain any secretory glands, the vagina is kept moist by cervical secretions (Waugh and Grant, 2006).

The external genitalia

These are also known as the vulva or pudendum and consist of the labia majora, labia minora, clitoris, hymen and vestibular glands (Waugh and Grant, 2006). The clitoris corresponds to the male penis and contains numerous sensory nerve endings. Stimulation of the clitoris has a role in sexual excitement (Tortora and Derrickson, 2009). The vestibular (Bartholin's) glands produce a small amount of mucus during sexual arousal, providing lubrication during penetration.

Breasts

The breasts are considered part of the reproductive system as they are required in order to provide sustenance for the infant. Breasts exist in males as well as females, but in a rudimentary form. In females, breasts develop at puberty under the influence of hormones, enlarge during pregnancy and lactation and atrophy in old age.

Within the breasts, clusters of milk-producing alveoli form lobules. The ducts from several lobules unite to form larger ducts which open on the surface of the nipple. The nipple lies on the outer surface of each breast surrounded by a pigmented area called the areola containing sebaceous glands to lubricate the nipple.

Sexual arousal in females

Sexual arousal is noted by erection of the clitoris and labia minora. Parasympathetic stimulation leads to these tissues becoming erect as they become engorged with blood. Breasts may also enlarge and the nipples become erect. Flushing of the skin may be present including the chest, breasts, neck and face. These changes are brought about by dilatation of blood vessels supplying the skin. Parasympathetic stimulation also causes the vaginal walls to exude a fluid which act as a lubricant. This fluid is added to by secretions from the Bartholin's glands.

During sexual intercourse the penis moves in and out of the vagina, leading to rhythmical contractions of the clitoris and vaginal walls. These contractions eventually produce stimulation that leads to an orgasm (climax) similar to that of the male. However, unlike males, females are potentially capable of experiencing several orgasms over a short period of time. As in males, during the sexual act a number of other physiological changes occur, notably an increase in heart rate and blood pressure, increase in respiratory rate and dilation of skin vessels.

Changes in the reproductive systems associated with ageing

Maintaining sexuality

The female reproductive system is the first to age naturally to the stage where it is no longer deemed functional. Menopause takes place over a period of several years, usually between the ages of 45 and 60 (Christiansen and Grzybowski, 1999). In comparison, some men can remain capable of complete reproductive function until the age of 80 or older. After this age, it is usual for an increased decline in male reproductive system function to the point where reproduction becomes less likely. The decline in sexual function in both men and women is related to a decrease in levels of sexual hormones (Christiansen and Grzybowski, 1999; Lueckenotte, 2000).

Sexual ageing is highly individual and there are many exceptions to the normal ageing patterns. Orgasm can be reached in both men and women into the ninth decade (Heath and Schofield, 1999). Indeed, some women have been known to have their first orgasm in their eighties (Heath and Schofield, 1999). Associated with ageing is a decline in the intensity of sexual desire and the need for sexual release as compared to younger individuals. However, sexual arousal continues to occur, but it can take longer for an older person to become aroused and to achieve orgasm. The four phases of the sexual response include arousal, plateau, orgasm and resolution. However, at times one of the phases may be omitted; for example, the person may become aroused but not attain orgasm (Heath and Schofield, 1999).

The ageing man

Testosterone

There is a decline in the production of testosterone with ageing. From the age of 45, testosterone is reported to decline at a relatively steady rate, and this change is due to the reduction in number and diminished responsiveness of the Leydig cells. However, as the kidneys do not remove all of the testosterone from the blood, the reduction in circulatory testosterone is limited (Christiansen and Grzybowski, 1999). Due to the steady decline in production of testosterone, serum androgen levels fall and reach their lowest levels in men aged over 70. This event is sometimes described as the andropause and is likened to the hormonal changes that occur in women during menopause (Wright, 2001).

Loss of testosterone is linked to ageing changes in the secondary sexual characteristics. It probably contributes to loss of muscle in the rest of the body and possibly contributes to a reduction in aggressiveness. The growth rate of facial hair slows but the hairs become more bristly so men continue to shave regularly. The vocal cords become thinner so that the timbre of the voice changes to a thin raspy quality (Christiansen and Grzybowski, 1999). Reduction in testosterone affects the penis so that it loses muscle tone and weight (Wright, 2001). There is also reduction in the size of the penis in relation to ageing changes. Loss of elasticity and contractility of the blood vessels affects the erectile tissue of the penis so that it becomes more difficult to obtain and maintain an erection during sexual arousal. Pubic hair becomes thinner and the testicles atrophy (Lueckenotte, 2000). Men over the age of 50 will undergo a decline in testicular mass. This reduction in testicular mass parallels the diminution in the number of Leydig cells. The Leydig cells may also become slower in their responses to LH.

Sperm production

The number of sperm produced diminish after the age of 50; their motility and viability also decrease. The total number of sperm produced by an average 65-year-old man is about 30% less when compared to a man of 25 (Christiansen and Grzybowski, 1999). However, men continue to maintain adequate amounts of sperm to fertilise an ovum into their eighties. The seminiferous tubules decrease in diameter due to an increase in the fibrous connective tissue of the tubular walls and the interstitial spaces, and this has a deleterious effect on the number of sperm produced. The secretions that constitute part of semen also decline with age. Even though the prostate gland increases in size, prostate secretion may decline significantly, along with the contractility of the prostate muscles that force the secretions into the urethra. The seminal vesicles decrease in weight after the age of 60 and their contribution to semen declines as well.

Changes in sexual arousal

There are a number of changes in sexual arousal that require some adaptation to remain sexually active. Men who are between the ages of 50 and 60 are usually satisfied with 1–2 orgasms per week (Heath and Schofield, 1999). However, after the age of 50, older men when compared to younger men require more direct and more intense sexual stimulation to achieve an erection and it takes longer for them to achieve an erection and ejaculation (Heath and Schofield, 1999).

The erection may be less firm and the angle of the erect penis tends to point to 90° as opposed to 40° when compared to younger men. Less ejaculate is produced due to a reduction in secretions from the bulbo-urethral (Cowper's) gland. Urgency for ejaculation decreases and may take longer to achieve. Orgasm may also occur but without ejaculation. Semen may seep out or is ejected into the urinary bladder. The frequency of penile contractions reduces during orgasm and semen is expelled with diminished force (Heath and Schofield, 1999; Wright, 2001). The testes no longer retract during orgasm. Once orgasm has occurred, the erection is lost rapidly and days may elapse before another erection can be achieved (Heath and Schofield, 1999).

The ageing woman

Hormonal changes related to the menopause

According to Christiansen and Grzybowski (1999), the ageing of the female reproductive system can be separated into two stages. The first being the menopause, which can be described as a period of quite concentrated ageing, and a gradual menopausal ageing where the menopause exerts its effect on the ageing body. Once a woman reaches the age of 45–50, only a few follicles remain which can be stimulated by FSH. Progressively, less oestrogen is produced and concentrations of FSH and LH rise. The falling concentration of oestrogen no longer acts as a feedback mechanism to prevent the rise of these hormones. These alterations occur before there are changes in menstrual cycle length and are a good predictor of the onset of an imminent reduction in reproductive ability. These changes are also a good indicator that the menstrual cycle will soon become irregular.

Once the peri-menopause begins and irregularity in the menstrual cycle occurs, decreasing responsiveness to the positive feedback effects of oestrogen becomes apparent (Wise, 2003). The normal fluctuating female cycle eventually stops and ovulation ceases. Corpora lutea are no longer formed and FSH and LH levels continue to climb associated with a lack of oestrogen and progesterone feedback. Surges in LH produce a response by the adrenal glands, with the release of adrenal androgens and cortisol. The release of these hormones together with the reduced levels of oestrogen may be linked with some of the features associated with the menopause as outlined in the following:

- Depression.
- Fatigue.
- Hot flushes with extreme flushing of the skin.
- Sensation of suffocating and dyspnoea.
- Irritability.
- Anxiety and mental disturbances that sometimes develop into psychoses.

Approximately 15% of women require treatment for symptoms associated with the menopause. This usually involves oestrogen replacement therapy, often in combination with progesterone. This treatment is referred to as hormone replacement therapy (HRT).

Effects of the hormonal changes on the female body

There is little circulating oestrogen remaining in the body once menopause occurs, and it is this loss that triggers a number of ageing changes. The ovaries shrivel and thicken with fibrosis, the ligaments and ducts of the breasts degenerate due to the loss of oestrogen and progesterone. The secretory cells in the breasts are not replaced due to the reduction in progesterone. The breasts therefore shrivel, sag and become pendulous. The ovarian ducts, uterus, vagina and external genitalia all reduce in size. Blood flow to the vagina decreases so that the lining of the vagina thins and loses much of its flexibility. The vestibular glands produce fewer secretions resulting in less lubrication during sexual intercourse which may become painful due to the loss of vaginal secretions and lubricants. Vaginal pH becomes more alkaline so that there is an increase in vaginal infections in older women as the vaginal secretions do not have the same antibacterial effect as in younger women. When comparing the types of vaginal infections found in younger and old women, infections among younger women are more likely to involve yeasts, whereas in older women infections involve bacteria that are not usually pathogenic in the hormonally supported vagina. There is a loss of fat in the mons veneris (pubis) which is the fatty tissue present in women above the pubic bone, thinning of pubic hair, shrinkage of the labia majora and thinning of the labia minora leading to exposure of the clitoris (Wright, 2001).

After menopause, significant calcium loss occurs linked to the increased activity of osteoclasts that are normally kept under control by the presence of oestrogen. Up to 2.5% of the body's calcium can be lost each year for the first few years after the menopause. However, this rate slows over time. Oestrogen also seems to have a protective role against atherosclerotic changes in the body; therefore, the reduction in oestrogen levels also increases the risk of atherosclerosis-related diseases. Reduction of oestrogen contributes to the thinning of the skin and the depletion of subcutaneous fat.

Post-menopause oestrogens are produced mainly from the adrenal glands. Adrenal androgens are also produced there and these are responsible for the development of male characteristics. The female voice may drop in pitch, facial hair appears, pubic and cranial hair becomes sparser while some hairs become coarser. There may also be a redistribution of fat around the abdomen.

Sexual arousal in older women

The strength of an orgasmic contraction decreases and the orgasmic phase is shortened (Lueckenotte, 2000). During orgasm, the vagina becomes less responsive and the number of contractions reduces to about half that of younger women. However, these changes do not interfere with sexual pleasure (Wright, 2001).

As with other organs of the body, there is decreased blood flow to the genital area in women as they age. Related to a decrease in genital blood flow is impairment in the vaso-constrictive responses during arousal (Heath and Schofield, 1999). The consequence of this is a lack of protection from penile thrusting which can lead to urethral and bladder trauma, increasing the risk of UTI. The clitoris decreases in size and breasts become less engorged during sexual arousal.

Sexuality in older people

Sexuality encompasses a number of factors including sexual health, sexual acts and body image. In 1975, the World Health Organisation defined sexual health as 'the integration of somatic, emotional, intellectual and social aspects of sexual being, in ways that are positive, enriching, and that enhance personality, communication and love' (WHO, 1975, p. 2).

The Royal College of Nursing (2000, p. 2) defined sexual health as 'the physical, emotional, psychological, social and cultural wellbeing of a person's sexual identity, and the capacity and freedom to enjoy and express sexuality without exploitation, oppression, physical or emotional harm'. Whereas Nay (1993, p. 199) defined sexuality as 'referring to the socially constructed roles, behaviours, identities and processes – prescribed and prohibited, enacted and avoided, admitted and denied, valued and devalued, relational and non relational – associated with female and male eroticism, reproduction, sex acts, thoughts, feelings, beliefs and attitudes. It refers specifically to those aspects of sensual, psychosocial and physical stimuli and responses associated with the pleasures and pains, fulfilments and humiliations of the person in the name of sex. It is broader than but included the acts of sex and being male or female'.

How we dress and how we feel about ourselves is also expressed in our sexuality. This also includes our relationships with others and how we communicate with those around us.

Sherman (1999) identifies the range of feelings and activities that can be included under the headings of sexuality and sensuality from the deepest longings for mutual affection to the simple enjoyment of the company of a loved one. Sexuality also includes a range of behaviours – touching, caressing and cuddling, genital intercourse with mutual orgasm and feelings of closeness and being wanted and valued as a human being (Sherman, 1999). Maintaining sexuality is one of the activities of living identified by Roper et al. (1996) and it is therefore a legitimate concern for nurses and other health-care professionals, and as such becomes part of their role to assess and manage the sexual health of the patients under their care. It is not only a legitimate concern for nurses, the nurse may be required to start any discussions about sexual health and sexuality as it may be difficult for patients to initiate this discussion (Taylor and Davis, 2006).

The expression of sexuality for older people varies from individual to individual. Numerous factors may influence an older person's views, desires and needs in relation to sexuality. Some of these influences include:

• The degree of sexual activity in earlier life.
• The enjoyment and fulfilment derived from sexual activity from past experiences.
• How the person feels about changes in physical appearance in relation to the ageing process and changes in sexual response.
• How the person feels about seeking sexual activity in later life.
• Feelings of embarrassment or guilt about aspects which society generally might not condone, such as masturbating, using erotic stimuli or the services of professional sex workers.
• Particular difficulties in later life, for example, monotony in a relationship, unresolved grief, seeking new partners, uncertainties about sexual performance.

(Heath, 2002)

Older people continue to have the same sexual desires as they did when they were younger, the ageing process does not affect this. The availability of potential partners may impact on the level of sexual activity, especially among people aged 85 and over as the census in 2000 identified that there are 4 men for every 10 women in this age group (Bancroft, 2007).

Although the ageing process influences both male and female sexuality, by far the biggest problem associated with sexuality and older people is societal attitudes towards this issue. Societal attitudes affect both an older person's willingness to share thoughts and problems about their sexuality and also the nurse's understanding and willingness to discuss this with older people. This can be seen when common myths and stereotypes associated with sexuality and older people are explored.

Younger people find it difficult to accept that older people continue to be interested in sex no matter their age. The society that we live in emphasises the importance of having youth and beauty together so that being physically attractive is an important component in sexual relationships. Given that the societal emphasis is on youth and beauty, we should not be surprised that younger people find it difficult to appreciate how older people can find each other attractive (Russell, 1998). We often find it difficult to accept that our parents and our grandparents may still be sexually active (Sherman, 1999). In addition, older people may have been brought up to think that sex should not be talked about and it therefore tends to be a taboo subject (Russell, 1998). Therefore, there may be situations where older people find it difficult to talk about the subject of sexuality and where nurses find it difficult to introduce it.

The whole issue of sex and old age is very rarely considered in the same sentence, although there is no doubt that there is an increasing willingness to bring it into the public domain. Sherman (1999) states that if the topic arises then we tend to use euphemisms such as intimacy rather than sex or sexual intercourse. Often the activity of living, maintaining sexuality, is changed to body image in care plans. Under this activity, comments such as 'likes to wear lipstick' is often noted rather than actually attempting to discuss the issue of sexuality. The words 'passion' or 'desire' and 'making love' are rarely used in the context of older people.

Societal attitudes towards sexuality in older adults often re-enforces the idea that all sexual activity ceases in middle age. If older men continue to remain sexually active, they are likely to be labelled as dirty old men, while women who continue to have an active sex life are labelled as nymphomaniacs. If men continue to express an interest in sex they are viewed as lecherous, whereas sexually active older women may be described as mutton dressed as lamb if they do not conform to the stereotype of how an older woman dresses and acts (Heath, 2002).

Heath (2002) goes on to state that older men can be described as handsome and distinguished, whereas older women are very rarely described as having these attributes (Heath, 2002). This is evident in the media where older men continue as anchor people for news programmes while older women are usually removed from this role in middle age. When older people marry later in life during their seventies and eighties, this becomes newsworthy as does fathering a child when a man is in his seventies and eighties. The misperception that surrounds older people about sexual activity is that they cannot or do not engage in sexual intercourse once they become old. However, the evidence suggests that older people continue to be sexually active into their eighties and nineties, but the frequency of sexual intercourse falls in old age. There are also some advantages for women post-menopause as they do not have to concern themselves with the risk of pregnancy. This can add to their sexual experiences and enjoyment of sex without the possibility of becoming pregnant (Peate, 2004).

There are consequences to ignoring the sexual behaviours of older adults. For instance, sexually transmitted infections including gonorrhoea, HIV and AIDS are rising rapidly among older people (Gott, 2006). Gott also states that divorce and remarriage rates in later life are increasing steadily, and there is a developing trend among older people to have intimate but non-cohabiting relationships. Past legislation may impact on older peoples' perceptions of sexual activity. It was only in 1967 that the Sexual Offences Act legalised homosexuality between consenting adults, and a number of older people who are gay or lesbian remember the period of time prior to the introduction of the legislation. Older people have tended to hide their non-heterosexual lifestyles although they are now becoming more open. The evidence suggests that health professionals do not discuss safe sex messages or even consider sexually transmitted diseases (STDs) as a risk factor for older people. Without such advice the number of sexually transmitted infections is likely to increase.

Sexual health in older people has been a low priority in government policy, practice and research (Gott, 2006). Older people and sexuality has not been considered in the

National Service Framework for Older People published by the Department of Health in 2001 (DH, 2001a) nor is there any discussion in the National Strategy for Sexual Health and HIV (DH, 2001b). However, there is a shift in attitudes and the topic is increasing in priority slowly. There are a number of reasons why this is occurring as outlined in the following:

- There is more willingness to talk about sexuality and the medical treatment of problems associated with sexuality.
- Increasing availability of medications to enhance sexual activity or to correct erectile dysfunction.
- Older people who are now reaching old age have different attitudes towards sex and behaviours, and this is related to the increasing expression of sexual freedom that has developed since the 1960s.

If older people have a problem with sexual activity, they are now more likely to seek advice and expect treatment. Health professionals may therefore be required to discuss such previously 'taboo' issues with these more liberated and knowledgeable patients. However, there may still be older people who find it difficult to talk about sex and sexuality and they may continue to be concerned about how the health-care professional views them. Some older people may also be reluctant to talk about sex and sexuality as they may be concerned about being viewed as having sexual desires and needs at their age (Gott, 2006).

Factors affecting sexuality in older people

There are a number of factors that can affect sexual function in older people. They include health issues, body image and prescribed medications. Some of the common health problems that can be directly linked to sexual dysfunction include depression, cardiovascular disease and diabetes. These diseases can lead to a decrease in sexual desire or affect sexual function adversely. Diseases can also have an impact on functional ability which can then affect sexual activity. This can involve either the patient or their partner. An example of this is osteoarthritis which limits the range of movement. This could necessitate sexual experimentation and consideration of body positioning during sexual encounters. Sexual intercourse need not be the only outcome, and other ways of attaining sexual satisfaction can be explored. Body image also needs to be considered in relation to an older person's sexuality. If an older person is viewed as asexual, their body image may be ignored by health-care professionals, for example dealing with changes in body image following surgery in the older adult may not be considered as an important part of their recovery process.

Older people are prescribed a variety of medications that can affect sexual function. This includes some anti-hypertensives, antidepressants, medications to reduce cholesterol, antipsychotics and seizure medications. Older people should always be informed that the medications that they are taking may have an effect on sexual function. Cognitive impairment does not prevent sexual desire, but it may complicate its expression (Wallace, 2008).

Point for Practice

Sara and Jacob have just celebrated their diamond wedding anniversary. Jacob who has been becoming increasingly frail is to be admitted to a residential/nursing home. How might the staff in the home help Jacob and Sara meet their need to express their sexuality?

Assessment of sexual function

The PLISSIT model was developed in 1976 by Jack Annon, an American psychologist. There are four levels of intervention in this model:

- Permission.
- Limited information.
- Specific suggestions.
- Intensive therapy.

The goal of assessment using PLISSIT is to collect information in such a way that the patient is allowed to express his or her sexuality in a safe environment and where they can feel at ease discussing any difficulties associated with their sexual activities (Wallace, 2008). The assessment should be completed in a private area, free from disturbance and where others cannot overhear the dialogue. The environment should be prepared in such a way that the older adult feels safe, comfortable and able to communicate freely with the health-care professional. It is important that the health-care worker ensures that their behaviour is non-judgemental and non-critical. The assessment should be carried out in a manner that is respectful to the client and in a way that conveys an understanding of an older person's sexuality. The health-care worker should never laugh or look surprised at the patients' responses.

Permission giving

The permission giving stage is the first step of the process and includes assessment of sexual function. Nurses must be willing to introduce the topic which will allow them to identify the patients' needs. As discussed previously, patients may be embarrassed by initiating discussion about their sexual activity; therefore, the nurse may need to begin the dialogue by giving the patient permission to discuss their sexual activities. This will reassure the patient that discussion about sexual activity is a legitimate remit of the nurse and therefore a reasonable topic of conversation. The patient thus has the opportunity to discuss any concerns.

There may also be opportunities prior to the permission giving stage where information in the form of leaflets and posters can be made available in waiting areas which promote services in relation to sexuality. The nurse may be unable to distinguish between patients who wish to discuss their sexuality or sexual health needs from patients who do not unless the matter is approached on an individual basis. There are many opportunities in primary health care and in the acute setting for giving permission. However, although nurses are giving permission to patients to discuss their sexuality, they are also giving patients the opportunity to refuse to discuss this topic. Wallace (2008) suggests asking the following questions to introduce the subject:

First of all, the nurse should ask a question in the form of seeking permission, for example, 'Would it be alright if I ask you a question about . . .?' Asking permission enables the patient to feel in control of the situation.

Other introductory questions can include:

- Many of my patients have problems with their sexual health as they age. Would it be alright if I ask you questions about your sexual health?

If the patient agrees, the nurse can follow up with further open-ended questions, for example,

- What concerns you about your sexual health?
- What changes have you noticed in your sexual feelings or functions since you were first diagnosed or treated for your disease?

Then the nurse should follow up these introductory questions by progressing to more specific questions. If permission is given by the patient, and it is appropriate, there is no reason why the partner should not be included. Any issues relating to sexual dysfunction in your patient may well have a negative effect on their partner.

Limited information stage

Stage two reflects the role of the nurse in giving information. The information may take the form of discussing the impact of an illness or treatment on the patient's sexual function. Nurses can also clarify any misinformation that the patient has. Any opportunities to dispel myths in relation to sexual health and function should be taken, and any factual information which could be construed as within the remit of the nurse should be offered. Information should also include education about the normal changes in sexual health related to the ageing process (Wallace, 2008).

Specific suggestions stage

The third stage involves a problem-solving approach which will help to meet specific needs of the older adult identified through previous discussion. This approach can include advice such as taking pain relief prior to sexual activity, if required, and trying different sexual positions if problems with movement are apparent. Advice in relation to body image can also be offered to help with older adults who may have issues with their perceptions of their body.

Intensive therapy stage

The final stage is more for health professionals who have undergone further education in relation to sexual health and sexual function in older adults, that is, those who have had specialist training in this field. Few nurses have sufficient training to provide intensive therapy and they therefore need to be aware of their limitations and direct the client to an appropriate health professional or services. This may include direction to see a psychotherapist (Wallace, 2008), appointments at genitourinary medicine (GUM) clinics, if required, and use of charitable organisations such as Help the Aged and Age Concern where specific advice is readily available (Taylor and Davis, 2006). Behaviour modification is also available for patients who demonstrate hypersexuality that may be linked to cognitive impairment (Wallace, 2008).

Management of health issues related to sexuality

If an older adult has any sexual worries or concerns, they may first approach a nurse for advice. Nurses must be aware that their attitude to this approach may influence the outcome of the discussion. Patients will be sensitive to others attitudes, feelings and responses to their questions and dialogue. Expressions of discomfort or disgust will be readily identified and discourage the person from further contribution. Sexual problems such as erectile dysfunction should never be discussed as a simple consequence of growing older.

Peate (2004) identified a list of practical tips that a nurse can offer to support the patient in these circumstances:

1. If a patient has any concerns about their sexual health, then they should contact their practice nurse or raise the issue with the nurse caring for them.
2. They should find out what possible side effects there may be of the medicines that they are currently taking. It may be necessary to consider changing medication if the drug is implicated in any sexual dysfunction.
3. They may need to alter positions when they have sex.
4. If dryness is a problem, they may wish to think about using a water-soluble lubricant.
5. If they tend to tire as the day goes on, then they may want to think about engaging in sexual activity in the morning.
6. If they have been provided with pain relief, they may want to take some prior to sexual activity to provide some pain relief.
7. Sexual intercourse is not the only way of experiencing sexual pleasure; they may want to try touch or massage.
8. They should be advised to relax and enjoy the sexual encounter, make sure that they have enough time without interruptions.
9. Older people should be advised to use safe sex techniques, for example, condoms if they are unfamiliar with their partner.
10. They must not assume that because they experience difficulties during sex, that they can't have a healthy sexual life.
11. Too much alcohol prior to activity inhibits, not enhances performance.

(Peate, 2004)

Summary

We hope that this chapter has caused you to rethink sex and older people. Too often in the popular psyche sex is seen as something that only the 'beautiful young' have any interest in. The reality is of course very different from this misperception.

In this chapter we have looked, in detail, at how ageing affects sex and sexuality. We have examined the physical and physiological changes that occur with ageing.

We have gone on to explore the issue of HIV/AIDS as it relates to older people. The evidence makes clear that HIV/AIDS is an issue for older people. Not only are people who developed HIV/AIDS now living into older age, but older people are also at risk of acquiring HIV/AIDS. We cannot provide the necessary care and advice that older adults need unless we first acknowledge that HIV/AIDS is an issue for this population.

References and further reading

Bancroft, J.H.J. 2007. Sex and aging. The New England Journal of Medicine 357(8), 820–822.

Christiansen, J. and Grzybowski, J. 1999. An Introduction to the Biomedical Aspects of Aging. McGraw-Hill, New York, NY.

Department of Health. 2001a. National Service Framework for Older People. DOH, London.

Department of Health. 2001b. National Strategy for Sexual Health and HIV. DOH, London.

Gott, M. 2006. Sexual health and the new ageing. Age and Ageing 35, 106–107.

Heath, H. 2002. Sexuality and later life. In Heath, H. and White, I. (Eds). The Challenge of Sexuality in Health Care. Blackwell Science, Oxford.

Heath, H. and Schofield, I. 1999. Healthy Ageing: Nursing Older People. Mosby, London.

Lueckenotte, A.G. 2000. Gerontologic Nursing. 2nd ed. Mosby, St. Louis, MO.

Nay, R. 1993. Benevolent Oppression – Lived Experiences of Nursing Home Life. School of Sociology, University of New South Wales, Sydney.

Peate, I. 2004. Sexuality and sexual health promotion for the older person. British Journal of Nursing 13(4), 188–193.

Roper, N., Logan, W. and Tierney, A. 1996. The Elements of Nursing: A Model for Nursing Based on a Model for Living. Churchill Livingstone, Edinburgh.

Royal College of Nursing. 2000. Sexuality and Sexual Health in Nursing Practice. RCN, London.

Russell, P. 1998. Sexuality in the lives of older people. Nursing Standard 13(8), 49–53.

Seeley, R.R., Stephens, T.D. and Tate, P. 2005. Essentials of Anatomy and Physiology. 5th ed. McGraw-Hill, Boston, MA.

Sherman, B. 1999. Sex, Intimacy and Aged Care. Jessica Kingsley Publishers, London.

Taylor, B. and Davis, S. 2006. Using the extended PLISSIT model to address sexual healthcare needs. Nursing Standard 21(11), 35–40.

Tortora, G.J. and Derrickson, B.H. 2009. Principles of Anatomy and Physiology. 12th ed. John Wiley & Sons, New Jersey.

Wallace, M.A. 2008. Monitoring functional status in hospitalised older people. American Journal of Nursing 108(4), 64–71.

Waugh, A. and Grant, A. 2006. Ross and Wilson Anatomy and Physiology in Health and Illness. Churchill Livingstone Elsevier, Edinburgh.

World Health Organization. 1975. Education and Treatment in Human Sexuality: The Training of Health Professionals. WHO Technical Report Series No. 572. WHO, Geneva.

Wise, P. 2003. The female reproductive system. In Timiras, P. (Ed). Physiological Basis of Aging and Geriatrics. 3rd ed. CRC Press, Boca Raton, FL.

Wright, L.K. 2001. Altered sexual patterns. In Maas, M., Buckwalter, K., Hardy, M., Tripp-Reimer, T., Titler, M. and Specht, J.P. (Eds). Nursing Care of Older Adults: Diagnoses, Outcomes and Interventions. Mosby, St. Louis, MO.

Chapter 11

Sleeping

Aims

After reading this chapter you will be able to discuss the normal sleep–wake cycle and identify strategies for promoting sleep in older adults.

Learning Outcomes

After completion of this chapter you will be able to:

- Describe the normal components involved in the regulation of the sleep–wake cycle
- Conduct a comprehensive patient assessment of a client/patient's sleep pattern using appropriate tools
- Detail the changes in the sleeping patterns that are associated with ageing
- Discuss the management of altered sleep patterns that may occur in older adults.

Introduction

In this chapter we will consider the normal sleep cycle, including the stages and function of sleep. We will then examine how ageing may impact upon the normal pattern of sleep/waking. Accurate assessment of a person's sleep–wake cycle is essential prior to recommending interventions with a view to improving a person's sleep pattern.

We shall consider some problems associated with older adults' sleep quality. These include sleep apnoea, restless leg syndrome, insomnia and REM sleep disorders. A number of strategies that may aid sleep in older adults will be suggested.

The normal sleep cycle

Sleep is defined as 'a reversible behavioural state of perpetual disengagement for unresponsiveness to the environment' (Carskadon and Dement, 1994, p. 16). In the typical

The Physiological Effects of Ageing: Implications for Nursing Practice, First Edition
© Alistair Farley, Ella McLafferty and Charles Hendry
Published 2011 by Blackwell Publishing Ltd

adult, the total amount of sleep per day is ~7 hours (Timiras, 2003). Sleep progresses through a distinct number of stages which are repeated at ~90-minute intervals. Sleep wakeful patterns are regulated by the reticular activating system (RAS) found within the brainstem and the hypothalamus. Neurotransmitters also play a role in regulating sleep and wakefulness. When the RAS is stimulated, a state of consciousness or wakefulness is experienced. The RAS helps to maintain this state of wakefulness and is also involved in the changeover from sleeping to waking. Inactivation of the RAS produces the state of sleep (Tortora and Grabowski, 2004). The hypothalamus establishes patterns of wakefulness and sleep which are part of our circadian (daily) rhythms. Neurotransmitters involved in promoting and increasing levels of wakefulness include acetylcholine, norepinephrine and dopamine, whereas serotonin, melatonin and adenosine growth factors all promote sleep (Huether and McCance, 2004).

There are two distinct phases to the sleep cycle. One phase is referred to as non-rapid eye movement (NREM) sleep. The other phase is known as rapid eye movement (REM) sleep. These two phases of sleep can be differentiated by physiological characteristics.

Sleep begins with NREM state, which progresses through four stages. This phase is initiated when neurotransmitters are withdrawn from the RAS and arousal mechanisms are blocked (Huether and McCance, 2004).

- Stage 1 is preceded by a state of wakefulness but where eyes are closed and the person is generally relaxed. During stage 1 NREM, which is the lightest stage of sleep, the person is in a transitional period of drifting off to sleep. They are easily aroused during this stage.
- Stage 2 is a period of light sleep where the person becomes even more relaxed. If a person is wakened during this stage, they are aware that they have been sleeping. Body movements are less frequent during this stage and dreams begin, which can be recalled on wakening.
- Stage 3 NREM is the first stage of deep sleep where body movements are further reduced.
- Stage 4 NREM is the deepest and most restorative period of sleep, during which the person is generally quite still. Decreases in heart rate, blood pressure, respirations, temperature and metabolism occur during this stage. Muscle tone is also decreased. Arousal from stage 4 NREM sleep requires intense external stimuli.

Stages 3 and 4 are sometimes called slow-wave sleep because slow waves are demonstrated on an electroencephalograph (EEG).

The four stages of NREM sleep are followed by REM sleep. The deepest level of relaxation occurs during REM sleep which is also known as paradoxical sleep as EEG activity is similar to the pattern during wakefulness. REM sleep is associated with bursts of REMs under closed eyelids and dreaming. During the first episode of REM sleep, the REMs may be absent. Respirations, pulse and blood pressure fluctuate, are irregular and frequently elevated during REM sleep.

A typical sleep cycle consists of NREM 1 followed by NREM 2, 3 and 4 with possible drifting back through previous stages of NREM 3 and 2 before the REM stage begins. The NREM stage accounts for 75–80% of total sleep while REM accounts for 20%. Approximately 60 minutes into the sleep cycle, the REM phase begins and typically six cycles of NREM to REM sleep activity occur every night (Timiras, 2003).

Ageing changes with sleeping associated with the sleep–wake cycle

The main aim of sleep is to rest the body and the mind (Bunten, 2001). Indeed, sleep is very important in the maintenance of health. A number of factors relating to sleep are influenced by the ageing process, and these influences need to be considered when nursing older people. As people become older, sleep becomes more broken. More than 50% of people over the age of 65 living in the community and more than 66% of people living in long-term care report some difficulties with their sleep pattern. Sleep disorders not associated with the ageing process also become increasingly common with advancing age. Ageing changes that influence the quantity and quality of sleep need to be separated from actual sleep disorders, as it may be difficult to differentiate between the two. Other common complaints regarding sleep patterns include difficulties in falling asleep. One in three women and one in five men are affected by a delay in the onset of sleep (Bunten, 2001).

Ageing changes in the RAS may alter sleep patterns and also alter alertness and behaviour. These changes may be due to alterations in the production of neurotransmitters such as serotonin and melatonin, both of which enhance sleep.

With older age, there is a reduction in the amount of slow-wave sleep which is common during stages 3 and 4 of NREM sleep. There is also a decrease in the absolute and relative amount of REM sleep which makes it more difficult for older people to recall dreams on arousal (Linton and Matteson, 1997).

The total amount of sleeping does not necessarily change much with ageing. The main difficulty is related to sleep during the night being interrupted. This night interruption leads to the need to spread sleep time more widely over the 24-hour period. This is achieved by the addition of short naps during the day (Timiras, 2003).

Linton and Matteson (1997) suggest that total sleep time may decrease slightly but because older adults wake frequently during the night and spend longer time awake during the night, they may actually spend a longer time in bed. Older people are considered light sleepers as the transition between sleep and wakefulness is usually sudden.

There may be problems associated with falling asleep at the beginning of the night (sleep onset delay), and this seems to be influenced by changes in the circadian rhythms. Older adults may also go to bed earlier in the evening, but they also tend to rise at an earlier time in the morning (Wolkove et al., 2007a).

Accompanying the ageing process is a change in the distribution of REM sleep throughout the night. The first REM sleep commences earlier during an older person's sleep as the time spent in NREM sleep is reduced. Periods of REM sleep following this are usually equal in length during the night instead of increasing in duration, which is the pattern commonly seen in younger people.

There are major changes in the stages that constitute NREM sleep. Stage 1 NREM sleep seems to lengthen so that older people are more easily roused during this stage by sounds, touch and light. Fragmentation of sleep occurs due to disturbance in this stage. The changes in this stage seem to affect older men more than women; therefore, older men have an increased number of awakenings. There are also changes in stages 3 and 4 of NREM sleep where there is a reduction in both amount and depth of the sleep. There may also be a near absence of stage 4 NREM sleep.

The changes in the quality of the REM stage and stages 3 and 4 of NREM sleep adversely affect the efficiency of sleep for older people. The marked shortening of these stages may result in older people complaining that they have had little sleep during the night, although they have remained in their beds for the usual length of time. This may also explain why older people are more easily awakened than younger people. There also appears to be a cumulative reduction of sleep time at night so that about 40% of older people complain of insomnia (Timiras, 2003).

As described earlier, feeling sleepy during the day or taking more naps during the day may be an issue for some older people. However, not all older people take naps during the day, but the people who do may be trying to add to their total sleep time if they are unable to sleep satisfactorily during the night and awaken feeling unrefreshed. Older people may also nap more, simply because they have the opportunity to do so. Sleeping during the day may also be related to boredom. Napping does not seem to replace night-time sleep but rather supplements total sleep time. Naps of less than an hour in length do not seem to affect the person's sleep that night, but they do increase the person's levels of alertness during that particular day.

Acute sleep problems in the older adult can develop into chronic sleep-related problems which can include insufficient amounts of sleep over time, frequent and prolonged nocturnal awakening and persistent day sleepiness. It therefore becomes necessary to carry out a full and comprehensive assessment of a person's sleeping patterns and habits. Following this, a tailored management programme can be initiated to help alleviate and overcome some of these problems. In this way, acute episodes of sleeping difficulties may not develop into chronic issues.

Factors contributing to sleep pattern disturbance outwith the normal sleep–wake cycle:

- Sensory impairments such as visual or hearing difficulties can make it more difficult to interpret and respond to environmental cues. These cues can include time of day, levels of light and general activity level in the surrounding environment, all of which may help guide activity/rest patterns.
- Signs and symptoms of illness or disease that may interfere with sleep include paroxysmal nocturnal dyspnoea where the person develops breathing difficulties during the night which causes them to awaken, orthopnoea where the patient has to sit upright in order to alleviate breathing difficulties, anxiety, any experience of pain, sleep apnoea and having to rise in order to micturate (nocturia).
- Psychological stress can interfere with sleeping patterns. Stress can result in a reduction in sleep as the individual may worry over issues at night (McConnell and Murphy, 1997), which disturbs the normal sleep cycle. Dreams and nightmares can also disturb the normal sleep cycle.
- Grief and depression can interfere with sleep, either by causing difficulty getting to sleep or early morning awakening.

Changes in the physical environment can result in a change in sleeping habits, including a change to the normal pre-sleep rituals. Moving rooms, moving house, admission to hospital can all affect a person's sleeping habits, where the physical properties of the sleeping area may be different to the person's norm and pre-sleep rituals are disturbed. Noise levels, light levels and unfamiliar smells can all interfere with sleeping patterns.

If in hospital, it should be noted that nursing care practices at night can also interfere with sleeping whether directly related to the individual or another.

Many drugs including beta blockers, diuretics, corticosteroids, carbidopa, caffeine, nicotine and alcohol can all contribute to insomnia in older adults (Wolkove et al., 2007a). Alcohol can act as a relaxing sedative agent when consumed in moderation before sleeping, but night-time awakening can be a problem with moderately high blood alcohol levels due to sympathetic activation (Schoenfelder and Culp, 2001). Alcohol consumption also leads to the need to void. Withdrawal from medications used to induce sleep including hypnotics and sedatives or alcohol withdrawal can also precipitate insomnia (McConnell and Murphy, 1997).

There are a number of common features of sleep pattern disturbance:

- Complaints of difficulty in falling asleep.
- Awakening before or after the desired time.
- Disturbed sleep.
- Generally feeling tired.
- Feeling irritable.
- Restlessness.
- Disorientation.
- Lethargy.
- Dark circles under the eye.
- Mispronunciation and use of incorrect words.
- Frequent yawning.

(Adapted from McConnell and Murphy, 1997)

 Point for Practice

Consider older adults in a residential or nursing home setting. What measures might you employ to ensure good sleep hygiene in your clients?

Assessment of sleep

Assessment of older people's sleep patterns should include a thorough sleep history. Questions should include the following areas:

- Ask the person to describe a typical night's sleep.
- Identify how well the person functions during the day? This can include asking about daytime naps and how they feel as the day progresses.
- Identify any prescribed or over-the-counter drugs taken and typical alcohol intake (many of these can interfere with sleep).
- Ask if the person uses sleep-inducing medications.
- Identify the usual time of going to bed.
- Ask how long the person feels they lie awake before falling asleep.
- How many times does the person feel they awaken during the night? Is this in relation to any symptom of disorders such as breathing difficulties, pain, nocturia or palpitations? Dreams or nightmares may precipitate more frequent awakenings.

- Identify the normal time for awakening in the morning.
- A sleep diary can be kept for several weeks to help identify sleep patterns – this can be particularly helpful.

(Adapted from Linton and Matteson, 1997)

Other questions to consider asking include:

- Do you experience any problems in staying asleep?
- Identify how the person rates their quality of sleep.
- Identify if the environment affects quality and quantity of sleep. Has the sleeping environment changed of recent?
- Are caffeine containing beverages consumed after late afternoon?
- Is a night-time ritual followed before retiral for the night?

(Adapted from Roach, 2001)

Personal beliefs about sleep should also be explored as the person may place much importance on an arbitrary number of hours sleep each night (McConnell and Murphy, 1997). When assessing a person's sleep patterns and habits, the nurse should also remember to consult family members and seek their input and assistance.

As use of medications increase with age, including over-the-counter medications and prescription drugs, it becomes important to take a careful drug history which includes both these categories of drugs (Roach, 2001). Older people may be more susceptible to the stimulatory effects of some chemicals including caffeine, the stimulatory effect of which can be as much as 8–14 hours. The effects of caffeine may be even more pronounced in older adults due to possible decreased liver function impairing caffeine clearance.

Schoenfelder and Culp (2001) suggest that a visual analogue scale (VAS) may be useful when assessing the quality of sleep in older adults. This scale works along the same lines as the VAS associated with assessing pain which most nurses will be familiar with. Such scales, for example, require the person to place a mark on a 100-mm horizontal line that ranges from one end for the best sleep ever to the other end with the worst sleep ever. The distance of the mark along the line is then measured and this can be compared to other night's sleep.

Sleep disorders in older adults

Apnoea

Sleep apnoea is a common disorder amongst older adults. Obstructive sleep apnoea is an upper respiratory disorder where the upper airway is repeatedly obstructed during sleep, which reduces airflow – hypopnoea or stops it – apnoea (Wolkove et al., 2007a). Sleep apnoea therefore involves interruptions to breathing during sleep. Relaxation of the pharyngeal muscles during sleep causes the tongue and palate to fall backwards resulting in an obstruction of the airway. These obstructive incidents result in interrupted, poor-quality sleep, nocturnal oxygen desaturation and a considerable reduction or absence of REM sleep (Wolkove et al., 2007a). This sleep disorder is far more likely to occur in overweight men. A pattern of loud snoring followed by varying lengths of silence is typical of this condition and any comments or changes in sleep patterns, including episodes of loud snoring made by partners should be followed up.

Periods of apnoea or hypopnoea (cessation or slowing of respiration) increases with age from an average of five disturbances per night at 24 years of age to about 50 per night at the age of 74 (Timiras, 2003). Apnoea results from a collapse of muscles in the upper airway resulting in a total airway blockage. This typically lasts for around 10 seconds and is reversed on wakening, where the upper respiratory muscles regain their activity. Hypopnoea is a partial blockage of the upper airways where the amount of oxygen entering the lungs is considerably reduced. Again, this episode typically lasts for around 10 seconds before the person wakes up and begins to breathe normally again. These incidents account for the disturbed sleep experienced by many older adults. This disturbance to the night's sleep contributes to tiredness, drowsiness and fatigue the next day (Wolkove et al., 2007a), which has been shown to increase the risks of falls and involvement in road traffic accidents (Timiras, 2003).

Leg movements during sleep

Sleep-related leg movements during sleep are also common in the older adult. The prevalence of leg movements when sleeping increases with age. Thirty-three per cent of older people experience twitches or leg discomfort every two to three times, every minute during much of the night. These movements often lead to a brief arousal from sleep and they appear to be related to loss of coordination between motor excitation and inhibition (Timiras, 2003). As with sleep apnoea, these movements disturb a night's sleep which leads to daytime drowsiness and fatigue in many older adults.

Restless leg syndrome is a very different sleep disorder from periodic leg movement disorder described earlier. Patients with restless leg syndrome can experience tingling, unpleasant cramps and painful sensations before the onset of sleep. These are usually felt in the lower extremities. A crawling feeling under the skin is also described. When the symptoms occur the person is likely to move or massage their legs. Typically, these symptoms are experienced not long after getting into bed and contribute to a delay in sleep onset. This syndrome occurs in ~10–35% of people over 65 and is more likely to occur in women compared to men (Wolkove et al., 2007a). The onset of this condition appears to be linked to a reduction in dopamine production and administration of levodopa or dopamine agonist can decrease the symptoms associated with this disorder.

Insomnia

Insomnia is defined as difficulty in falling asleep with episodes of wakening during the night followed by difficulty in falling asleep again (Mauk, 2006). Insomnia affects ~50% of all older people, with older women more likely to report greater difficulties in falling asleep when compared to older men. Insomnia in women may be linked to a reduction in the hormone oestrogen post menopause (Roach, 2001).

Roach (2001) identifies two categories of insomnia in older people. They are:

1. Transient insomnia.
2. Chronic insomnia.

Transient insomnia is normally a temporary condition where the sleep problem is related to a situation which increases stress levels. Examples of stressful situations include admission to hospital, financial concerns, health worries, bereavement or grief. The insomnia is commonly self-limiting and should resolve relatively quickly, lasting no more than 5–7 days. Medication is not usually necessary; however, if it is required, then hypnotics or sedatives should not be prescribed and administered for longer than 2–3 days and the smallest effective dose possible should be given.

Chronic insomnia normally lasts much longer than transient insomnia. It is described as a sleep pattern disturbance that has been present for more than 1 month. This category of insomnia is associated with the additional symptoms of anxiety, irritability, fatigue and impaired mental functioning (Roach, 2001).

There are a number of reasons why insomnia is common among older people.

Frequent awakenings during the night may also be related to medical conditions. Common and well-recognised causes of insomnia include depression and anxiety disorders. Older adults are particularly at risk of depression related to, for example, the loss of a partner, social isolation, underlying disease and onset of dementia.

Adults with dementia are prone to sleep disturbance and those diagnosed with Alzheimer's disease are especially likely to have sleep disturbances. Not only is dropping off to sleep difficult, but regular and frequent episodes of wakening through the night are also experienced. It is not unusual for these sleep disturbances to increase in their severity as the dementia progresses with sufferers also sleeping for longer periods throughout the day. Agitation is common especially in the late afternoon and evening where symptoms such as confusion, disorientation and restlessness are experienced. These can result in inappropriate vocalisations, expressions of violent behaviour and a tendency to wander. These symptoms are collectively referred to as 'sundowning' relating to the time of day when they are first expressed.

Insomnia is common in patients with Parkinson's disease (PD) who may also experience frequent awakenings with difficulty returning to sleep. However, adults who are diagnosed with PD also commonly experience vivid dreams, nightmares and leg jerks, all of which upset a night's sleep.

Other factors including retirement which results in a change of routine and which may utilise less energy during the day can lead to insomnia as an individual may be in the process of transforming from a more active work lifestyle to a more sedentary retired lifestyle. This alone may lead to an abrupt change in demand for daily physical activity and energy and can lead to change in demands for sleep. Until adjustments are made, the individual may suffer from insomnia.

REM sleep disorder

REM sleep disorder commonly affects people over the age of 60. Dreaming usually occurs during REM sleep. At this time, voluntary muscles are normally inhibited which prevents typical skeletal muscle movement during dreaming. However, REM sleep disorder is typified by the loss of this normal muscle inactivity so that there is an increase in movement at this time. During REM sleep disorder, the person may engage in a number of different body movements some of which can be forceful and damaging to either themselves or their bed partner. It is possible for the person to get out of bed and walk about. They may also thrash their arms and legs while in bed, and it is this range of movement that put partners at risk of being kicked or punched. Ninety per cent of older people who suffer from this condition are men (Wolkove et al., 2007a), and it is often linked with neurodegenerative disorders including PD, multiple sclerosis and Alzheimer's disease. Interestingly, where PD is concerned, REM sleep disorder may be a precursor to the development of Parkinson's as it may be present for a number of years before the signs and symptoms of PD are obvious (Wolkove et al., 2007a).

General interventions

When identifying appropriate interventions relating to sleep disorders for older people, changes associated with the ageing process need to be taken into consideration. The sleep patterns of older people differ from those of younger people for the reasons already identified (McConnell and Murphy, 1997). However, older people continue to require the same amount of sleep but it may be distributed differently over a 24-hour period when compared to younger people and this may include the need to nap during the day (Roach, 2001). Roach also identifies that sleep requirements may increase with advancing age. Therefore, it is important to explain to older people the ageing changes and how they will influence their sleep pattern.

Interventions should be implemented after a thorough sleep history has been taken. The aim of the nursing interventions should include:

- A decrease in the overall length of time spent in bed.
- A reduction in the number or frequency of naps.
- Advice relating to re-organising the structure of daytime activities and increasing day-time energy levels to enhance sleep at night.
- Education on the use of relaxation techniques.
- A combination of all of the above.

The outcome of nursing interventions is therefore to promote sleep in older people in such a way that they will awaken refreshed and energised. There are a number of simple measures that can be implemented to achieve this outcome.

Nursing interventions should include informing older people of normal ageing changes associated with sleep. The environment should be modified to provide ambience that is conducive to sleep. The room that is being used for sleeping should not be too warm; however, it should be kept above 60°F. The bedclothes and pillows should be kept clean and comfortable. It is also recommended that the bed is only used at night and activities that occur in bed should be restricted to sleep and sex (Linton and Matteson, 1997).

Exercise should be actively encouraged at any time during the day within limits of level of the person's mobility. Roach (2001) suggests morning or early evening exercise, and Linton and Matteson (1997) suggest afternoon or early evening as times for exercise. Increasing levels of daytime activity should encourage an individual to feel pleasantly tired and sleepy at night. Naps during the day should be reduced or avoided although this may be difficult to achieve if normal sleep patterns are being redistributed.

It is useful for older people to try and follow a similar sleep routine each night, so that the individual goes to bed at approximately the same time each night and rises at approximately the same time each morning. These practices are known as developing good sleep hygiene. Additionally, older people should develop sleep rituals to try and aid sleep. The rituals can include having a warm bath, taking a light snack before bedtime or drinking a glass of warm milk. Warm milk aids sleep as it contains a substance called tryptophan which acts as a natural sedative. Tryptophan enhances production of melatonin produced by the pineal gland. Melatonin promotes and enhances sleep.

There are a number of relaxation strategies that may be useful to add to the sleep ritual to try and improve sleep patterns. These include meditation, visualisation, music or reading a book at bedtime (Roach, 2001). If an individual awakes during the night, they should be encouraged to engage in monotonous activities to try and induce sleep again. The concept of counting sheep probably falls into this category. If falling back to sleep continues to be a problem, then the following advice should be given.

If an individual cannot sleep after 10–15 minutes of lying awake, then they should use diversionary strategies to try and aid a return to sleep. Diversionary strategies include turning on the light so that the individual can read or watch television until they feel sleepy again. Additionally, it is important to rise from bed at approximately the same time each morning in order to promote a regular pattern that supports the circadian rhythm (Linton and Matteson, 1997).

Advice should be given to older people regarding both caffeine and alcohol intake. Caffeine is a stimulant and should therefore be avoided after 5 pm or at least 3–4 hours before bedtime. Alcohol in moderation often causes sleep disturbances in that an older person will fall asleep but they are often awake during the night as the sedative effects of alcohol wear off. Moderate to high alcohol intake may also lead to the need to rise in order to void. Alcohol should therefore be limited to no more than one drink prior to going to bed.

Medications to promote sleep whether they are prescribed, that is hypnotics or sedatives, or over-the-counter sleeping aids should be avoided or used for no more than 2–3 days as they can cause rebound insomnia. Rebound insomnia is the inability to fall asleep or stay asleep after discontinuing medications to help with sleep.

Benzodiazepines have traditionally been the most commonly prescribed hypnotics for use by older people. They work by depressing stages 3 and 4 of NREM and REM sleep and by increasing stage 2 NREM sleep. However, if there is a requirement to prescribe and administer hypnotics, the starting dose should be half the dose prescribed for younger people. Remember that ageing changes reduces the efficiency of the liver in metabolising drugs. These drugs can cause increased daytime sleepiness and a lack of motor coordination leading to a reduction in mobility, an increased risk of falls and subsequent fractures and a decreased ability to carry out activities of living. Older people therefore need to be monitored for these unwanted effects if they are prescribed these groups of drugs. There are other possible side effects including confusion, forgetfulness, wandering at night, paradoxical agitation (where an opposite reaction to the medication occurs such as restlessness and agitation after taking a sedative) and differing levels of cognitive impairment (Wolkove et al., 2007b).

If the person is admitted to hospital or long-term care, a number of issues need to be taken into account. In hospital, the patient should be encouraged to adhere to their normal sleep rituals as much as possible. Any symptoms that make sleep more difficult such as pain or breathlessness should be managed appropriately. Staff should plan to have minimum disruptions during the night (Roach, 2001).

In institutional settings, effort should be made to consolidate all nursing activities in order to reduce the number of interruptions to patients who are asleep. When patients are checked hourly overnight, interventions should be made when patients are awake. However, if a patient has been sleeping for three rounds of checks, they should be wakened if they require nursing interventions. In this way, a patient's night's sleep is disturbed as little as possible within an institutional setting.

Specific interventions

Staff should note how much sleep individuals actually achieve during the night. Patients who are suspected of having sleep apnoea should have their oxygen saturation levels monitored during the night (McConnell and Murphy, 1997). Patients should be advised to sleep upright or on their side to reduce the risk of sleep apnoeic episodes. If overweight, then weight loss is advisable.

Continuous positive airway pressure is a method of respiratory ventilation which has been used to treat sleep apnoea. This method of ventilation delivers a stream of compressed air which keeps the pharyngeal airway open, thus preventing airway obstruction. By adjusting the applied air pressure appropriately, the airflow acts as a pneumatic splint. Patients are required to wear a nose or full-face air mask which many older adults have difficulty in accepting, especially if the person has to rise in order to void as they must then remove and reapply the air mask each time they rise. Compliance can be improved by educating the person how to carry out this procedure (Wolkove et al., 2007b). The use of sedatives or hypnotics is not recommended for older adults who have sleep apnoea.

Phototherapy in the form of evening light therapy may be effective for early morning insomnia. Use of evening light can increase total sleep time, REM sleep and slow-wave sleep, all of which contribute to a good night's sleep and increase the likelihood of the person waking up feeling refreshed. Evening light exposure may also help some patients with Alzheimer's disease by helping to reduce disturbances to their sleep–wake cycle.

Summary

Sleep – all of us know and appreciate the value of a good night's sleep. However, for many older people, getting a good night's sleep seems elusive. In this chapter, we have identified a number of problems that may prevent the older adult from sleeping well. We go on to consider a range of strategies that may be employed to improve the quality and quantity of an older person's sleep.

Health-care professionals who work in residential or other institutional settings need to give careful thought to how the environment may or may not be conducive to sleep. All health-care professionals should be familiar with the concept of good sleep hygiene and how they may promote good sleep hygiene in their clients/patients.

References and further reading

Bunten, D. 2001. Normal changes with aging. In Maas, M., Buckwalter, K., Hardy, M., Tripp-Reimer, T., Titler, M. and Specht, J.P. (Eds). Nursing Care of Older Adults: Diagnoses, Outcomes and Interventions. Mosby, St. Louis, MO.

Carskadon, M.A. and Dement, W.C. 1994. Normal human sleep: an overview. In Kryger, M.H., Roth, R. and Dement, W.C. (Eds). Principles and Practice of Sleep Medicine. 2nd ed. WB Saunders, Philadelphia, PA, pp. 16–25.

Huether, S.E. and McCance, K.L. 2004. Understanding Pathophysiology. 3rd ed. Mosby, St. Louis, MO.

Linton, A. and Matteson, M. 1997. Age-related changes in the neurological system. In Matteson, M., McConnell, E. and Linton, A. (Eds). Gerontological Nursing: Concepts and Practice. 2nd ed. WB Saunders, Philadelphia, PA.

Mauk, K.L. 2006. Gerontological Nursing: Competencies for Care. Jones and Bartlett Publishers, Sudbury, MA.

McConnell, E.S. and Murphy, A. 1997. Nursing diagnoses related to physiological alterations. In Matteson, M., McConnell, E. and Linton, A. 1997. Gerontological Nursing: Concepts and Practice. 2nd ed. WB Saunders, Philadelphia, PA.

Roach, S. 2001. Introductory Gerontological Nursing. Lippincott, Philadelphia, PA.

Schoenfelder, D.P. and Culp, K.R. 2001. Sleep pattern disturbance. In Maas, M., Buckwalter, K., Hardy, M., Tripp-Reimer, T., Titler, M. and Specht, J.P. (Eds). Nursing Care of Older Adults: Diagnoses, Outcomes and Interventions. Mosby, St. Louis, MO.

Timiras, P. 2003. The nervous system: functional changes. In Timiras, P. (Ed). Physiological Basis of Aging and Geriatrics. 3rd ed. CRC Press, Boca Raton, FL.

Tortora, G.J. and Grabowski, S.R. 2004. Introduction to the Human Body: Essentials of Anatomy and Physiology. 6th ed. John Wiley & Sons, New Jersey.

Wolkove, N., Elkholy, O., Baltzan, M. and Palayew, M. 2007a. Sleep and aging: 1. Sleep disorders commonly found in older people. Canadian Medical Association Journal 176(9), 1299–1304.

Wolkove, N., Elkholy, O., Baltzan, M. and Palayew, M. 2007b. Sleep and aging: 2. Management of sleep disorders in older people. Canadian Medical Association Journal 176(10), 1449–1454.

Chapter 12

Final Thoughts on Ageing

Growing older – we are all in the middle of doing this right now. Even as you read this book you are ageing. Do you feel any different now than you did 1 hour ago? What about 1 week ago? Last year, or the year before?

Ageing is always with us and we may not give it much thought from one moment to the next. At some point or another we may say 'I'm not as young as I used to be!' Perhaps, climbing the stairs leaves us a little out of breath. Or maybe we notice more aches and pains after a day on the allotment than we used to.

It is important to remember that growing older is happening to everyone all of the time. Growing older is not a disease! Yes, growing older may be associated with a range of disorders but and this is an important 'but', most of us can expect to have a good quality of life as we age. Disease and infirmity is not a *sine qua non* of ageing. It is not inevitable.

Yes, there may be some activities that you can no longer undertake with advancing years, but not many. It may be that they take you longer, or that recovery needs more time. But remember, older people generally have more time. There are fewer deadlines, less pressure, life is usually more relaxed. Whilst some older people continue to work, most are retired or semi-retired. This allows for the pursuit of hobbies and interests that may only have been enjoyed fleetingly, if at all, when you were younger.

Yes, growing older may have its limitations and constraints, but it also has its freedoms and benefits. Look at how much more relaxed and less stressed grandparents often are with their grandchildren than they might have been with their own children. Old age is a time when many people give something back to their local community. Volunteering is very popular amongst older adults, such as visiting the housebound; helping at local schools, sharing history and traditions from days gone by; helping to care for a part of their local environment; being more involved in their faith community and so on. Many older adults take up or return to study, perhaps gaining qualifications that they did not have the opportunity to gain when younger.

Our older people are a rich resource for our communities, local and national. Many employers now look for ways to retain the experience and wisdom that their older employees possess.

The Physiological Effects of Ageing: Implications for Nursing Practice, First Edition
© Alistair Farley, Ella McLafferty and Charles Hendry
Published 2011 by Blackwell Publishing Ltd

It is true that for some, growing older may bring frailty and poor health. In this text we have provided, in detail, an insight into the physiological changes that ageing brings. We have presented a number of common health problems that are particular to older adults. We have done this so that the reader may make links between the physiology of normal ageing and ill health. We have endeavoured to include a wide range of age-appropriate health assessment tools in order that health-care professionals can make sound assessments of their older clients/patients. We have presented a number of strategies that should help to restore the individual to health, or at least, minimise the disruption that ill health may bring to an older person's activities of living.

Growing older may have its own unique challenges, but it is also a time of new opportunities. As health-care professionals, we have a duty to help our older clients face up to the challenges and maximise the opportunities.

As one now quite elderly and iconic gentleman was fond of saying – 'Live long and prosper!'

Index